Effective Communication Skills for
Health Professionals

Effective Communication Skills for Health Professionals

2ND EDITION

Philip Burnard PhD

University of Wales College of Medicine, Cardiff, Wales, UK

First published in1992 by Chapman & Hall

Second edition published in 1997 by Stanley Thornes (Publishers) Ltd

Reprinted in 2001 by:
Nelson Thornes Ltd
Delta Place
27 Bath Road
CHELTENHAM
GL53 7TH
United Kingdom

02 03 04 05 / 10 9 8 7 6 5

A catalogue record for this book is available from the British Library

ISBN 0 7487 3312 4

Page make-up by Columns Design Ltd

Printed and bound in Spain by GraphyCems

For Sandy Kirkman and Deb Salmon
and for Paul Morrison

Contents

Part Four Communication Through Teaching: Educational Skills

Acknowledgements

Many people have helped in shaping the way I have thought about the issues in this book. First and foremost, my family, Sally, Aaron and Becky, who have always been supportive despite my being so often caught up with the computer. Without them, I know I could not have written. Second, my colleague and friend Paul Morrison, from whom I learned so much and who now works in Australia, and another colleague and friend, Jim Richardson, who has offered useful and critical commentary on various ideas in this book as well as more general support and friendship. Finally, to Sandy Kirkman and Deb Salmon – to whom this book is dedicated – who have made me think more carefully about gender differences in communication and who have always been caring and supportive. They have also made me laugh more than most people.

Earlier influences should also be acknowledged. I learned a great deal in a short space of time from John Heron, an inspired teacher and thinker, and from Professor Peter Jarvis, who always had time and who was always positive and caring. Charles Bailey was another person who sharpened my thinking and encouraged me to learn, as did my friend Mark Avis, who continues to keep me on my toes. Another friend, Ian Spencer, always offers an alternative view of things and I always appreciate him for that. Finally, particular thanks to the publishing team, Rosemary Morris, Sally Champion and Serena Bureau, who were always accessible, patient and available at the right time.

About the author

Philip Burnard is Vice Dean of the School of Nursing Studies at the University of Wales College of Medicine in Cardiff, Wales. The author of a variety of books on communication, ethics, computing and counselling, he has also contributed more than 200 articles to health-care journals in different countries. He has studied the teaching of communication skills in the USA and Canada and has been a visiting lecturer in various countries around the world. In 1996 he was made a Fellow of the Florence Nightingale Foundation in recognition of his contribution to nurse education and to international relations. In 1996 he was a Visiting Fellow at various universities in Australia. His research interests include communication, counselling, AIDS counselling, forensic psychiatric care, interpersonal skills and experiential learning. Dr Burnard lives in Caerphilly, South Wales, with his wife and two children.

Introduction

We are all communicating, nearly all of the time. What we say, how we say it, what we wear, how we sit, how we write, the text that we send to others and so on: all of these things are aspects of how we present ourselves to other people. We may not be able to do anything about that. What we *can* improve is our *means* of communication. We can do much to improve the way we communicate. Consider the following situations.

- You are working with a colleague who is senior to you and whom you don't like very much.
- You are interviewing a teenage boy about his family.
- You are 'off duty' and having a drink with some of your colleagues.
- You are presenting a short paper to a conference on some research that you have just completed.
- You are asked to write a report on what you see as health-care priorities in your area.
- You are at home with the person you live with or with your family and a client rings to talk to you.
- You are at a meeting and you are asked to take the chair.
- You are preparing to write up a piece of research.
- You are posting a message onto the Internet.

In each case you are communicating but do you communicate easily and effectively in each of these situations? Which situation would be easiest for you and which would you try to avoid? Would you be 'yourself' in each situation or would you have to 'bluff' a little in some of them? This book is about the skills involved in coping with these and other health-care situations.

Effective Communication Skills for Health Professionals is about practical ways of enhancing communication between health professionals and their patients or clients and between colleagues. Its aim is to encourage you to think about how you present yourself to others in everyday life. There is no 'right' way, no single method of ensuring that you will be understood by others but there are many straightforward methods of helping you to communicate more effectively. This book highlights some of them and points to some obstacles that may get in your way.

WHO THIS BOOK IS FOR

Communication is a vital aspect of health care. Just look around you at your colleagues and notice whether they communicate effectively. More painfully, perhaps, look at yourself as you talk to patients, clients or colleagues. Most of us can benefit from a little self-analysis and a bit of rethinking about taken-for-granted aspects of how we come across to others. This book is for all students in the health-care professions and at all levels: in basic training or education, at diploma, graduate and postgraduate levels. It will be of use to doctors, nurses, occupational and speech therapists, physiotherapists, social workers and voluntary workers – anyone who is intimately involved in managing, caring for or working with others.

WHAT IS IN THE BOOK

The book focuses on clusters of skills which are identified under the following headings:

1. **Personal Skills:** individual communication		2. **Therapeutic Skills:** communication with clients
	THE HEALTH-CARE PROFESSIONAL	
3. **Organizational Skills:** communication with colleagues		4. **Educational Skills:** communication through teaching and learning

Medicine
Nursing
Occupational Therapy
Social Work
Physiotherapy
Counselling
Psychotherapy
Complementary Therapies
Speech Therapy
Dentistry
Voluntary Work

The first part of the book focuses on you as a health professional. It deals with aspects of self-presentation or what is sometimes called 'impression management'. Chapter 1 identifies a structured approach to improving writing skills. Assertiveness is addressed in Chapter 2 and the section closes with a chapter on a topic that underpins all the others: self-awareness.

The second part of the book focuses on therapeutic skills. Chapters 4 and 5 describe a range of listening and counselling skills. Chapter 6 is about running groups. Again, the emphasis in these chapters is on developing skills.

The focus of the third part is organizational skills. Senior health professionals (and, increasingly, more junior ones) all have to manage other people. How do you do it? Traditionally, many health professionals have never received training or education in management; they have tended to learn it by doing it. Chapter 7 looks at general management skills. Chapter 8 discusses the skills involved in managing meetings and the section closes with a chapter on interview skills.

Part Four opens with a chapter which discusses teaching skills and will be useful to anyone who has to teach colleagues or clients in any setting. Whilst there are a variety of philosophies of teaching and learning, many of the basic *structural* aspects of teaching can be identified easily. The approach taken in this chapter is concerned with adult teaching and learning.

In Part Five, presentational skills are addressed. Many health professionals find that it is only a matter of time before they are called upon to talk to a fairly large audience at a conference or presentation. This chapter explores ways of making such presentations effective. The skills involved here will also be helpful when you have to present cases or plans to colleagues or managers in various settings.

The final part of the book closes with a chapter on computers and computing skills: what to look for and what computers can do to make your communication more effective. It also discusses the Internet, probably the fastest growing aspect of communication that there is.

The last section of the book is a Communication Skills Questionnaire which you can use in one or more of the following ways:

- as a self-assessment and self-evaluation instrument before, during and after reading this book;
- as a means of identifying which skills you need to work on further;
- as a basis for discussion in group work.

The book closes with a detailed bibliography of further reading so that the themes in this book can be followed through.

HOW TO USE THE BOOK

The emphasis throughout the book is on three issues:

1.   the development of practical communication skills;
2.   the reader's growing awareness of their own communication skills;
3.   the issue of being *critical* about what is under discussion.

The aim is always practical. Theory and research are referred to and referenced throughout the text but the reader who wants more detail of any given concept or skill is referred to the detailed bibliography at the back.

You may want to read the book through at one sitting. More probably, though, you will turn to sections or chapters on issues that concern you in the present. Each chapter can stand on its own and describes and discusses specific skills. You can easily dip into sections of it.

At the end of each of the four sections, there is a skills checklist. These are to encourage you to reflect further on your own skill levels. They can also encourage discussion or disagreement. As I have noted above, there is no right way in human communication. The point, though, is to become increasingly aware of how *you* communicate and the effect you have on others when you do.

A point about language. I have tended to keep it personal throughout the book and refer to 'you' – the reader. I have also referred to the health professional as 'she' and the health-care recipient as 'he'. I am aware of the problems of sexism in writing but can find no better compromise at the moment. I have adopted the word 'client' to refer to any health-care receiver. Again, I appreciate that some people may prefer the word 'patient' or 'resident' or other descriptor. I feel that the word 'client' is far more straightforward to read than a lengthy 'client/patient/ resident' label.

In this new edition, I have tried to add more critical commentary and debate. Communication is a complicated process and the central issue of *meaning* runs right through it. What do people's utterances, writings and behaviours *mean*? This would seem to me to be an urgent issue for discussion. Also, I sense that I am more tentative in this edition. Certainly, I am much less certain about many of the issues under discussion than I was when I wrote the first edition. The world is changing rapidly and communication styles are changing with it. We communicate more readily with computers than we did five years ago. We have different theories to explain the way in which people communicate. I have tried to address some of these issues in this edition. Following comments from readers, I have also reorganized the chapters to make them flow in a more logical order.

Communication between people occurs on so many levels. First, there is the *linguistic* level. The fact that we have learned and used a language gives us a common bond with some people and not with others. Further, we *use* language in different ways. How I use a word may not necessarily correspond with how you use it. There is room, then, for misunderstanding. There is also room for a considerable degree of sharing of both ideas and feelings.

Second, there is that level of communication that tends to be called 'non-verbal' – all the bodily movements, gestures and so on that we use both consciously and unconsciously to express ourselves. The temptation sometimes is to believe that we can 'read' non-verbal communication in others according to some sort of formula. While this may occasionally be true, in many cases we use subtle and idiosyncratic forms of non-verbal communication to try and make ourselves understood. Just as we have our own vocabulary of words, phrases and meanings, so we have our own vocabulary of gestures and signs. Part of the process of understanding communication involves the appreciation and interpretation of other people's non-verbal behaviour at the *individual* level.

Third, we communicate in context. We are almost always communicating to particular people, in particular circumstances. While we are communicating, we are engaged in another complex process of trying to make sense of what other people think or feel about us. We are trying to assess the *impact* of our communication on other people and on the situation in which we find ourselves. The contextual element of communication draws on all sorts of complex features such as our cultural background, our beliefs and values and our sense of 'position' in the current situation. Communicating when we are in the role of 'patient' may be different to communicating when we are in the role of 'doctor'.

It is possible, too, to argue that we communicate beyond language and non-verbal levels – intuitively, perhaps. Although the mechanisms of how such intuition 'works' are unknown, it seems such a common feature of human life that we might do well not to dismiss it too quickly. David Lodge (1995) notes one of the quirks of age differences in people's understanding of other people. He describes how partners in a long-standing relationship no longer need to talk to each other so much. They know the other person so well that all sorts of understandings pass between them without words. However, as Lodge points out, this lack of need to talk is often interpreted, by younger people, as a sign that the partners have run out of things to say to each other. Silence, in the company of people who know each other really well, need not be interpreted as a sign of lack of communication.

Further, communication is not limited only to verbal and non-verbal forms. We communicate through the written word which itself takes many forms. We may write letters, we may use e-mail, we may write papers and books. All of these are forms of communication and, again, depend on factors such as language, vocabulary and context. What is missing from any written communication is the non-verbal element but this is often compensated for because the medium of writing is so different to that of spoken language. Thus, as you read this book, you may or may not form an impression of the writer that is or is not borne out when you meet the writer. In a sense, we may be 'different people' when we talk and write.

Both spoken and written communication benefit from being *clear*, *simple* and *structured*. If we are to communicate with others through speech or writing and if we are to be truly understood, then these three features seem vital. While it is often obvious that unclear and complicated *written* communication is not easy to read, a moment's thought reveals that *spoken* communication which is complicated is also difficult to understand. Also, the *structure* eases understanding further. These three principles are particularly important in the health-care fields which usually involve two people: a practitioner and a patient or client. Very often, the patient or client is in something of a subservient role in relation to the practitioner. They do not start (or continue) as real equals. If each is to understand the other, both will benefit from clear, simple and structured communication. This is not to suggest that the patient or client needs to be patronized or to have things 'simplified' for them but to note that just as clearly written prose is both easy and attractive to read, so clear verbal communication can strike home so much more directly to us.

I hope you will find the book useful and enjoy working through the activities. I hope, too, that you will take issue with some (but not all!) of the things I have written. The science and art of human relationships are still fairly new. We have a long way to go before we understand what happens when two or more people meet and talk to each other. In the meantime, as we care for other people, we can try.

Philip Burnard
Caerphilly, Wales, UK

Reference

Lodge, D. (1995) *Therapy*, Penguin, London.

PART ONE

Communication and the Individual:
Personal skills

Introduction

Communication starts with ourselves. When we set out to communicate with others, we first have to address that we, too, are human beings, with thoughts, feelings, beliefs, attitudes, prejudices and preferences. Before we meet others, we have, in a way, to meet ourselves. There is an increasing realization in the health professions that we must also care for ourselves. In the first part of this book, three elements of communication skill are examined. First, in Chapter 1, the question of how to improve writing skills is addressed. Whether we are writing essays and projects or reports for a management committee, we all have to write. Many academics are also required to write for publication. This issue is also explored in this chapter. Interestingly, expressing ourselves in written words can help us to express ourselves more clearly face to face. Someone once wrote that 'I don't know what I think until I hear what I say'; it may be an improvement, sometimes, to write out what you think, before you say it. Thus the first chapter starts with writing skills.

Chapter 2 is about being assertive. Assertiveness skills are not only important to enable us to care effectively for others, they are also the means by which our own needs are met. If our own needs are frequently ignored or bypassed we are on a course for burnout: the outcome of caring for others without paying attention to ourselves. On the other hand, there are, as we shall see, problems with assertiveness. Who defines what passes as assertive behaviour? Are there differences between male and female communication that preclude any attempt at generalizing about assertiveness? These issues are also addressed.

Chapter 3 is about that which underpins all aspects of caring and communication: self-awareness. With increased self-awareness we can learn to help others by staying in touch with our own thoughts, feelings, attitudes and beliefs. The chapter identifies practical ways of enhancing such awareness. It also treats as problematic the concept of self-awareness. After all, the notion is a complicated one and assumes that we have a clear, agreed understanding of what 'self' involves – which we do not. The chapter therefore includes a debate about some of the issues that surround notions of self.

Writing skills

1

AIMS OF THE CHAPTER

In this chapter, the following skills and issues are discussed.

- Basic principles of writing
- Keeping references
- Layout
- Writing essays, dissertations and theses
- Writing for publication
- Using a computer for writing larger projects

BASIC PRINCIPLES

Although health professionals face a variety of writing tasks, many of the rules of good writing apply to all. In this chapter we explore some of the principles of effective written communication. First, the accent is on identifying certain basic rules. Then the focus shifts to keeping references. Any health professional who has to undertake basic or further education will be required to reference projects, essays, dissertations and reports. It pays to think a little about how such references may be recorded. In the later parts of this chapter, the discussion moves on to the layout of a written piece and then on to report writing and writing for publication. Increasingly, the route to development in the health professions, for the career-minded person, is via published work, often, although not always, in professional journals. This is in itself a form of communication: the communication of new ideas and research to a wider audience.

What basic principles can be applied to all writing? A shortlist of such principles would include at least the following.

- Write short sentences.
- Write short paragraphs; three or four sentences is nearly always enough.
- Write to communicate, not to impress. Inflated language and extensive use of jargon rarely impress the reader. Nor do they usually impress editors and managers.

- Avoid lengthy quotations of other people's work. Wherever possible paraphrase the writing of others, giving full acknowledgement to the original writer in the form of a reference, for example (Brown, 1989).
- Write as you speak. Read through what you write and ask yourself: 'Would I *say* this?'. If you wouldn't, think about how you could rewrite what you have written to make it more readable. People often make the mistake of thinking that 'correct' writing somehow sounds more intelligent than 'readable' writing.

For many health professionals, particularly those who are working in education or doing courses, writing should become a habit. It is not a question of writing only when a piece of work is required. It is useful to get into a routine of writing. If you can, write every day, even if this means keeping a diary. Such a diary can easily be computerized. All you have to do is open a new file in a word processor and write descriptive pieces about what has happened that day. The whole process of writing – working with a word processor, shaping phrases and sentences, editing your work, saving files – will help when it comes to writing more formal pieces. The fact is that word processing can be tiring if you are not used to it so you need to keep in practice. You also need to keep in practice in the process of writing itself. Like most skills, writing skills improve over time.

In the current climate, it is also true that most health professionals can benefit from writing pieces for publication. These can range from short reports in weekly magazines, through articles in referred journals to books. Any published pieces are material for a CV and can benefit your career. This used to be the case only for those in an academic career but more and more it applies to anyone working in the health professions.

KEEPING REFERENCES

Many health professionals need to keep references to the books and papers that they read. The important thing is to develop a system of recording that suits you best and that you will maintain. Many people start a reference collection with good intentions only to discover that the whole thing becomes too cumbersome. As a general rule, keep the simplest records that you can but ones that will lead you straight back to the book or paper in question. The minimum that you will need to record for each item is:

- the name of the author;
- the year of publication;
- the title of the book or paper;
- the publisher (for a book) or the name of the journal (for a paper).

Many people collect their references in simple card files which are readily available at stationers, as are the cards that go with them. Also available are index cards to keep them in order. It is usually better to choose the 8″ × 5″ cards which allow for more detail to be recorded. A useful layout for a bibliographic reference card is this:

Author(s):	Year of
	Publication
Title:	
Publisher or name and details of journal:	
Location:	
Comments:	
Keywords:	

This card is then completed and filed alphabetically under author. In the comments section, it is possible to record keywords for cross-referencing the item with other items and to save important quotes. A completed card looks like this:

Author(s): Anderson, P.	Year: 1996
Title: Stress in communication	
Publisher or name and details of journal: Davis and Jones, London	
Location: Cardiff Central Library	

Comments:

This has a useful review of theories of stress. Takes a 'biological' view of stress rather than a psychological one.

> 'Talk of stress is endemic in the health professions. It is as though the concept was quite new and necessarily dangerous' (p 16).

Keywords: Stress, psychology, life sciences

Card files are not the only way of recording references. Some people prefer to keep them in an index book. This is rather like a home telephone directory with index pages sticking out of the side. As new references are found, they are written into the appropriate section and alphabetically, by author.

The other way of keeping references is to open a database on a computer. The advantage of this method is that as the list of references becomes larger, the computer database allows you instant access to particular items or sets of items. For example, you may want to find all your references under the heading of 'psychology'. Whilst you could work through each of your cards and pull out all the appropriate ones, the computer database can do it for you almost instantaneously. It can also help you to prepare reference lists at the ends of essays, projects, dissertations, theses and books. There is a range of specifically designed bibliographical database programs available, both commercially and as shareware. Shareware is software that is made available through a distributor for a nominal sum. You try it out and if you like it, you pay the author of the software a small payment. This represents a good way of trying out a bibliographical database to see whether or not you are going to get on with it. Bear in mind, though, that if you continue to use a shareware program, you must pay for it. On the other hand, you are usually free to pass shareware disks to friends and colleagues for them to evaluate the programs. This style of marketing is unique to computer software and, so far, operates without being moderated in any way.

EndNote Plus is an example of a commercially produced program for handling and storing bibliographical references. It works under *Windows* and allows you to insert references into the text that you are writing. It also enables you to draw up reference lists from those references, at the end of your piece. If you use the Harvard system of referencing and decide that you want to switch to the Vancouver, *EndNote Plus* will handle this too. Like all such systems, much depends on your own way of working. If you are methodical and likely to keep the bibliographical database completely up to date all the time, then a program like this may be invaluable to you.

The alternative is to use a standard database program such as *Access* or *Paradox*, though, in the end, this is likely to be a case of using a sledgehammer to crack a nut. Perhaps the most straightforward method of storing bibliographical references on disk is to keep them in a word-processing file. You keep a file especially for holding references and as you add new ones, you use the 'sort' function to put them all in alphabetical order. It is easy to search through such lists and find the references you want and it is also easy to cut and paste references out of the list for use in essays or other projects. This approach also means that you do not have to pay for a stand-alone database system. You simply use the word processor that you use for writing.

The other point about computers is that they can be used to *search* the literature. If you have access to a fairly large library, you will probably be able to search the literature via their CD-ROM system. If you have access to the Internet, you will also have 'free' access to bibliographical searching facilities such as MEDLINE. Most searching facilities on computer allow you to gather together huge quantities of references to the topic of your interest. Many searching facilities also allow you to view abstracts of papers and books. In this way, you can read a summary of the work before you decide whether or not you need to obtain the full publication. Once you have searched for references on a particular topic, you can download those references to disk, take the disk away with you and examine each of the references on your own computer. It makes sense these days to become familiar with computer referencing systems. First, the method of searching is relatively simple and can give you access to many references. Second, there are now so many journals published in almost every field that computer searching is the most logical approach to exploring what has been published in your field. Increasingly, too, journal publishers are making the full text of their journals available on the Internet. This means that you can now browse through complete journals as they are published and cut and paste important pieces. In this way, you can quickly build up a library of 'quotes' from journals that you find online.

LAYOUT

Any writing that you do needs to be organized. The time to think about such organization is before you start the writing. One of the most effective means of planning any writing project is through the use of *outlining*. These are the stages:

Stage 1 Brainstorming

In this stage, you write down, at random, any thoughts, ideas, hunches that you have about the writing project. Nothing is banned at this stage. The aim is to produce as many ideas as you can. Many you will not use in the project itself but, at this stage, the more varied and even bizarre, the better. The odder ideas can lead on to more practical ones. Once you have filled a page with jottings of ideas in this way, you identify the ones that you will keep and strike out the others. Then, you look for 'patterns' in the ideas that remain and group them together. Finally, you move on to the next stage, beginning to organize your ideas more formally.

Stage 2 Identifying Key Headings

Having identified some groups of ideas, the next task is to find headings for those groups. Those headings then serve as the sections of your project. It is helpful to aim at between five and ten headings, whatever the nature of the project. If you are writing an essay, the ten can be ten themes that you address. If you are writing a book, they can be ten chapters.

Stage 3 Identifying Subheadings

Next, you carefully work through the list of headings and fill in the subheadings and possibly, the sub-subheadings. It is rarely useful to break up your work into more than three sets of headings. Once you have completed this stage, all that remains is to allocate a word limit to each heading and subheading and then to write out the body of the text.

The whole process of outlining in this way is speeded up with the use of a word-processing package. Then, the headings and subheadings can be moved around at will and new ones added as necessary. There are also outlining programs specially written for this purpose. An excellent one that is released as shareware (see Chapter 3) is called *PC Outline*. It allows you to generate as many ideas as you wish and then organize them into a range of hierarchies. Alternatively, you may find the whole process easier with an A4 pad and a pen.

WRITING ESSAYS

As we have seen, the key to effective writing is to *structure* your work. This is particularly important when writing essays. It is sometimes tempting, when time is short, to sit and stare at the blank screen or the blank sheet of paper and to believe that an essay can be written in one go, from scratch. Structure, though, makes the seemingly impossible possible. The most mechanical method of writing an essay is to lay out the various headings and subheadings and then to 'fill in the gaps' between each of these. If you choose to work this way, you may find that you do not necessarily want to write the essay from the beginning. Instead, you may prefer to start with the part of the essay with which you are most confident, complete that and then go back and finish the other parts. Either way, you need to use headings and subheadings. They are not only the means of helping you to structure your work but they also help your reader to follow what you have written.

You also need to differentiate between those essays which are essentially *descriptive* and those that are also *critical* in their approach. Many lecturers and teachers insist, appropriately, that essays should contain critical commentary and it is worth distinguishing between these two.

A *descriptive* essay is one in which the writer identifies other people's work, writes about it and generally describes what is going on in the field. For example, the health-care student writing about counselling may first define it from the literature and then describe various theories of counselling. She may then go on to discuss the research that has been done in the field. Finally, she may end her essay with a summary of what has gone before.

On the other hand, the *critical* essay is one in which ideas are not merely described but are 'taken apart': the writer deconstructs or is critical of the theories and ideas of other people. Thus, in the case of the counselling essay, the writer may not simply identify the range of definitions of counselling in the literature. Instead, she puts them under a microscope, argues about them and, perhaps, offers her own summary of what counselling might be. Further, she is prepared to argue about the relative strengths and weaknesses of counselling theory and is ready to challenge the research that has been done. As a rule, it is easier to write a descriptive piece than a critical one. In the end, though, most people find it more useful to learn to write from a critical point of view. It not only challenges what other people have written, it also challenges the writer herself.

Health professionals doing higher degrees and postgraduate diplomas are often expected to write critical rather than descriptive essays. The critical element is worth working at and, in the end, it becomes a way of life. One way of developing this critical frame of mind is to continually ask of the writer whose work you are reading 'How do you *know* that?' or 'What *evidence* do you have for that?'. Alternatively, continually ask the question 'But is there *another* point of view ...?'.

Essays, like all other forms of academic work, have to be appropriately referenced, using the Harvard or Vancouver method, according to the convention of the college or institution. It is important to learn both methods in some detail. Most colleges or college libraries offer guides to referencing and these should be followed to the letter. Examiners encounter many scripts that have some aspect of the references missing. Sometimes this is a place of publication, sometimes it is a date. The point is to get all your references exactly right. This will pay major dividends if you want to get your work published. It will also pay dividends in the shorter term goal of getting higher marks. Many examiners mark down if the presentation of the essay is not up to the appropriate standard.

It is often a good idea to ask to see other people's essays as an example for the layout of your own. Lecturers sometimes keep examples of 'good practice' and these are helpful. On the other hand, for some people, this approach can raise anxiety levels in that the reader feels 'I could never write like that!'. Rest assured, though, that most people look back on their own work and think 'Was *I* able to write like that?'. This is the irony: even when we are highly anxious about our written work, we are often pleasantly surprised at our own ability, at a later date. Try to see what other people have written but try not to get drawn into conversations where other people tell you, in great detail, what they are planning or what they have already written for their current essay. This sort of process is much like the 'post mortem' that sometimes takes place as people leave an exam room: neither these nor detailed discussions about essays usually help the person who is anxious about their writing.

If you have real doubts about your essay-writing ability, ask if you can submit a draft of your essay. There are pros and cons here. If you do submit a draft, then you are likely to be compelled to include in the final work the comments made by the person who reads it. On the other hand, allowing a lecturer to read your draft can reassure you that you are on the right lines. Sometimes, but not always, it is helpful to ask another student to read your draft. Bear in mind, though, that some students have a vested interest in finding your own work less than satisfactory and that, as a result, they may be overcritical. In the end, though, the rule is to write *something*. Even if you are very nervous and unsure of your topic, train yourself to set aside some time every day or every other day to write. Do not leave your essay until the last minute. Writing, like many other things, is a skill and can be improved simply by the process of becoming familiar with it.

STYLE

Style in essay writing is a difficult thing to describe. It may be useful to try to differentiate between three types: the *heavily academic*, the *journalistic* and the *simple*. The heavily academic style is seen less frequently these days. It was characterized by the use of complicated language, convoluted grammar and lengthy sentences. It was seen by some as the 'clever' way to write. Some journals expected academic writing to be of this type and, by extension, some students felt that they had to emulate the style in their essay writing.

On the other hand, the *journalistic* style goes to the opposite extreme. Sentences and paragraphs are very short, the style is emotive and often characterized by more opinion than hard evidence and debate. It is suggested that it is probably best to avoid both these styles and instead use the *simple*. By simple, I mean that ideas and concepts are conveyed clearly and with precision. I mean, also, that the writer does not attempt to be 'clever' in their writing but concentrates, instead, on conveying ideas and argument. In writing, as in many things, simplicity is often close to genius. If ideas are worth conveying, you should avoid their being misunderstood. To write simply and clearly is a skill like many others. It takes practice and a lot of self-editing. In particular, it requires that the writer tries at all times to cut away superfluous language and to concentrate instead on brevity and clarity. Oddly enough, reading classic novels can help in the development of this sort of style. If you read the work of, for example, Conrad or Trollope, you find a simple style of writing that is nevertheless powerful and descriptive. Writing does not have to be complicated in order to reach its goal or its audience. To write simply, then, should be everyone's aim. This is not to suggest that writing should lack *depth* or *complexity* but merely to note that even the most complex ideas, if argued well, can also be argued simply and clearly. Plato wrote of complex ideas but his writing is as clear and fresh as if it had been written 20 years ago. And Plato was writing philosophy.

TITLES

Sometimes students may choose titles of their essays. This is certainly the case with dissertations and theses. Although there is some debate about the issue, it is probably best to choose a *descriptive* title and not a *journalistic* one. An example of a journalistic title might be *The Baby and the Bathwater: social workers' views of care in the home*. A more appropriate title might be one that more literally describes the content of the project: *A critical discussion of social workers' views of care in the home*. There are a number of reasons for this. First, if the work is published in any format, it will be listed in bibliographies. The more literal title helps the researcher to identify, from such bibliographies, whether or not this paper really is one that they are looking for. *The Baby and the Bathwater* may prove to be a distraction. Second, the title is less emotive. It conveys the idea that the writer has taken the topic seriously and is reasonably dispassionate about the issues contained in the paper. That is not to say that one should not *feel* passionately about any given topic but to note that essays and other sorts of academic projects should offer a reasonably balanced view. Clearly, this is not the last word on the subject. No doubt there are many lecturers in colleges and university departments who would prefer to see more evocative titles used. Be guided, though, by what is most frequently seen in the academic journals. Most of the titles in such publications are of the more descriptive type.

EDITING THE FINAL VERSION

There are certain issues to address before you hand in your essay. These concern the accuracy and format of the final version. There are certain conventions to observe in terms of layout (although there will be some 'regional' variations from college to college). As a rule, though, you should do the following.

1. Spell check the document when you have finished writing the essay.
2. Scroll through the essay on the computer screen and make sure that you have appropriate *paragraphs* in the text. It is generally a good plan to have at least two paragraphs to each page and sometimes three.
3. Double line space the document.
4. Use only a single type of *font* or typeface. The most frequently used font is Times Roman or a variant of it. The text that you are reading now is similar to a standard Times Roman font. At all costs, avoid the use of 'fancy' or unusual fonts.
5. Embolden headings throughout the text and make sure that this is consistent. Generally, emboldening has replaced underlining in computer text. In an essay between 2000 and 5000 words long it is probably best to use only one type of subheading throughout the essay.
6. Make sure that the pages are numbered.
7. Write a clear and simple front page for the document. This page need only contain the name of the college, the name of the course, the title of the essay and your name. Again, this should be typed bold and in the same font as the body of the text. You do not need to use larger or more complicated fonts for this cover page.
8. Always read through the final, printed-out version of the essay. While you will have checked it (and you may have used the grammar checker) on screen, it is widely acknowledged that it is quite easy to miss typographical and other errors while reading from the screen. The final, 'hard' copy is the one to read through carefully. Check, too, for any errors the word processor has introduced, such as shifts in spacing, irregular margin sizes and large gaps between words. These, too, are easily missed when scrolling through on the screen.

9. Print out the appropriate number of copies to be handed in and print out a further copy for yourself. This will make life easier if you are asked to discuss your work with a tutor.

10. *Always* make a backup copy of your essay. Even if you keep your essay on your hard disk, you *must* have a copy on a floppy disk. This is an immutable rule of computing. Hard disks break down. If yours does, you are likely to have lost your essay and any other work that is on your hard disk. Always make backups: this is the first and last rule of computing. If you do not heed it, you will live to regret it.

WRITING DISSERTATIONS AND THESES

There is an increasing demand for Master's degrees and courses which lead to the award of a PhD. While not everyone will want to continue their education to these levels, many health professionals do. For most Master's degrees, the student is expected to produce a dissertation while for all doctoral degrees (save those in some courses involving music or dance) the student must produce a thesis. It should be noted that in North America these terms are reversed: a Master's project is known as a thesis and the final report of doctoral work is called a dissertation.

Master's dissertations tend to range from 20 000 words in length for students who do a 'taught' Master's to about 60 000 words for those who do a Master's degree by research. The latter types of courses often lead to the degree of Master of Philosophy. The word limit for a PhD thesis is often 100 000 words. It is important to know the limitations laid down by your particular institution. It is also important to know whether or not *minimum* numbers of words are specified. If you are required to write a dissertation of up to 20 000 words, you may not be allowed, for example, to submit a dissertation of *under* 15 000. Such matters should be clarified before you start.

WRITING FOR JOURNALS

Many health professionals write for journals and magazines. Many more do not because they think that they could never get anything accepted for publication. On the other hand, others feel that an essay they have written for a course might make a good published article. It might, but there are better ways of doing things.

Writing for journals and magazines involves ensuring that you are very familiar with the publication you are writing for. So the first stage in getting into print is selecting the right journal. There are two approaches to the second stage. Some people feel that it is best to write a letter to the editor outlining the proposed article. Others feel it is best to send off the manuscript and let the editor decide on its strengths and weaknesses. I think the second way works better. The letter approach takes up more time and you may be asked to write a paper that was quite different to the one you had in mind.

On the other hand, if you choose to send the manuscript off directly, then you must make sure that it *exactly* fits the requirements of that journal. All professional journals publish 'instructions to authors', usually at the back of each copy. Follow these to the letter. If you slip up on any one of the requirements, many journals will simply return your manuscript. Therefore, if the instructions ask for two manuscript copies, double line spaced, on one side of A4 paper, send just that. Also send a covering letter stating that what you are sending is original and is not being offered to any other journal.

Never send duplicate copies of a manuscript to a variety of journals. What will you do if it is accepted by two? Also, some journals do not send out proofs for checking by the author. In this case, you risk the same paper being published in two journals. Attractive as it may sound, this is a sure way of encouraging editors never to take your work again.

When you send a manuscript off to a referred journal, it will be sent 'blind' to one or more professional referees. The 'blind' here refers to the fact that your name will not be on the manuscript when the referees receive it. That way, they cannot be prejudiced by knowing your name.

After the referees or the editors have made a decision, you may be asked to rewrite part of the paper. If so, do it exactly in the way that has been suggested. The reviewers and the editor know best. Also, make the alterations as quickly and as accurately as you can.

Alternatively, your manuscript may be accepted outright. With acceptance may come a letter offering you a fee on publication of the article. You can haggle over this figure but it is best to accept it in the early stages of your writing career. If you have submitted your work to a referred journal, it is unlikely that you will be paid for your work but a published article in a referred journal is usually a welcome addition to your CV.

WRITING BOOKS

Many health professionals would like to write a book. Whilst the whole process of book writing cannot be addressed here, the stages involved can. The secret to writing a book, particularly one that is non-fiction, is *structure*. The more organized you can be the better.

Stage 1   The Idea

First, you need to make sure of two things. Do you have enough to say to write a book? Is there a market for what you want to write about? If you are unsure about the answer to the first, careful planning at the proposal stage can help. If the answer is then 'no', you may want to consider writing a book jointly with a colleague, partner or friend. Alternatively, you may want to edit a book written by a collection of experts, including yourself. If the answer to the second question is 'no', then it is unlikely that a publisher will give you a contract to go ahead and write the book. Notice the order here: first a contract, then the book. Do not write the book first and then try to find a publisher. You may feel that the book is very good (and, of course, it may be) but the publisher may want quite a different sort of book. The publisher is also much more likely to know about the market for the sort of book that you want to write.

Once you have identified exactly what it is you want to write about, contact a commissioning editor of a publisher and send them your proposal. It is reasonable practice only to submit a proposal to one publisher at a time. Also, the process of having a proposal reviewed can take some time. Most editors will send it to one or more experts in the field who then often take some time in sending back their verdict.

Stage 2   The Proposal

The proposal is a vital part of the book-writing process. It shows the publisher exactly what you have in mind and also helps you to organize your ideas and plan your work. Most proposals for most publishers look very similar and the following is a useful format.

- *Title*. Whilst you may agonize over this, it need not be binding. Either you or the publisher may suggest changes at a later date.
- *Your name, qualifications, job title and address*. Remember to include your phone number and offer both home and work addresses.
- *Rationale*. Here, you justify the writing of the book you have in mind. Try to keep this to about two paragraphs but choose your words carefully. This section may make or break your proposal.
- *Market*. Most publishers will expect you to have identified, fairly carefully, the particular market that you have in mind. The process of identifying this market is also a very good way of deciding upon the 'level' that you will be writing at.
- *Comparison with other titles*. Find three or four other books in your field and write a short summary of each of them. Then write a note about how your proposed book will improve upon or supplement these books.
- *The author*. Here, you sell yourself. Write a short résumé of your professional life to date. Your main aim here is to convince the editor that you are both an expert in your topic and also able to write the book.
- *Contents*. Write out the titles of the chapters and under each, offer some subheadings to indicate the content. Don't forget to start with an introduction and finish with a bibliography and index.
- *Number of words and illustrations*. A fairly standard short textbook is between 50 000 and 70 000 words long. This one is about 65 000. You need to indicate your upper word limit and stick to it if you are offered a contract. Illustrations of any sort are expensive. Very few publishers will want you to include colour or monochrome photos. Some will ask you to prepare the artwork for any

diagrams that you include. It is best to keep diagrams and illustrations to a minimum. The cheapest sort are 'word illustrations' which show blocks of words surrounded by straight lines.

• *Date of submission of manuscript.* People write at different speeds. Even so, the publisher will want to know that you will not be writing your book forever. Given that the process of getting a contract can take some time, it is useful to suggest 'submission of manuscript one year from signing of contract' or a figure that seems reasonable and appropriate to you. A book of about 50 000 words should take between 6 months and a year to write.

Take some time over the preparation of your proposal. It is often the only link between you and the publisher and it is the document that usually decides whether or not the company will go ahead and commission your book.

Stage 3   The Contract

Once the commissioning editor has received your proposal, she will send it off for review by one or more experts on the topic. Four things can happen after this (and sometimes some considerable time after this – things do not happen quickly in the book trade).

First, the editor may write back and say that your proposal has been accepted by the company and that you will shortly be receiving a contract. This is unlikely if this is your first book.

Second, the editor may ask you to amend your proposal along the lines suggested by one or more of the reviewers. If you accept this, make the amendments and send back the proposal.

Third, the editor may ask for a sample chapter. If this happens, take your time over it. You don't have to write the first chapter. Write the one that you are likely to be most comfortable with and write it well.

Finally (and this is the worst option) the editor may thank you for your proposal but suggest that the company cannot take it on at present. This is a polite way of saying that your proposal has been rejected. Some publishers will give you details about why it has been turned down, others will just turn it down. Either way, pick yourself up, print out a new copy of the proposal (or make modifications to it) and send it off to another publisher. If it is also rejected by them, consider writing another book. Don't give up!

If you are successful, you will be sent a formal contract to read and sign. Read it carefully and make sure that you understand and agree with all of the clauses. If you are in doubt about anything in it, contact the editor and ask for clarification.

Stage 4   The Writing

The easy part is over: now for the writing. As noted above, structure is the thing that will help in the writing of a book. You will already have planned out your chapters when you prepared the proposal. Now elaborate on those basic outlines. If you are working with a computer, open up separate files for each chapter and lay out an outline of headings and subheadings. This will make the whole thing seem much more manageable and help to ensure that you don't repeat yourself.

Next, set yourself a plan of working. Try to write regularly and attempt to complete a certain number of words every week. If you want to be professional, write something every day even if you don't feel like it. The discipline is good, your writing is likely to improve and you will get the book written. Remember, too, that you don't have to write the whole book in chapter order. You may decide to write the most difficult chapters first or start with an easy one and then take on an awkward one.

However you decide to write, the three rules that apply throughout the writing process are:

- be accurate;
- be concise;
- be consistent.

Stage 5   The Checking

Once you have written the first draft (and you may find it easiest to do this at speed, particularly if you are working on a computer), read through the whole manuscript, critically. Rewrite and polish as necessary. Pay particular attention to ensuring that you have used short sentences and paragraphs. If possible, ask someone else to read it and comment on it for style and readability. Finally, check all the spellings, diagrams, page numbers and references. Some of the things to look out for in the final read-through are:

- spelling errors;
- errors of punctuation;
- repetitions of the same word in a sentence;
- split infinitives (although there is a continuing debate about whether or not this is so important);
- long words;
- sexist expressions and phrases;
- clumsy and awkward phrases;
- lengthy sentences and paragraphs.

Print out a final draft, double line spaced and on good quality paper. Make sure that all the pages are numbered (at this stage of the business, the publisher will refer to them as 'folios': 'pages' refer to *printed* pages). Have two photocopies made of the manuscript and send the original top copy and one photocopy to the editor. Keep one photocopy for yourself. Even though you should have the manuscript on computer disk, the chances are a subeditor will call you with some points that need checking. It is always easier for both you and the subeditor if you can go straight to the printed page. The printed copy will also make life easier when you have to answer the list of queries that the subeditor sends you later in the process.

Stage 6   The Waiting

Next, the wait. If the manuscript looks as though it satisfies the contract, the editor sends it out for reading. Sometimes it will go back to one of the reviewers who read the proposal. Such reading and commenting takes time and always longer than you think. If you are asked to rewrite sections or even chapters, do so. Again, the editor is likely to know more than you about the processes of writing and publishing. At some point, you will be sent a list of queries by the subeditor. This is the person who has to work slowly through your manuscript and try to make it publishable. This means that they may want to suggest changes of style or grammar. The subeditor will also pick up errors, inconsistencies and missing references. No matter how carefully you have checked your final draft of the manuscript, you will still find that the subeditor has unearthed mistakes. It is vital to the publishing programme that you respond to these queries promptly and clearly. The subeditor's queries will usually consist of a list of questions, with space next to each for your response. It is really important that your responses are unambiguous and cannot be misread or require further elaboration. It is not sufficient merely to write 'OK' next to a query or to tick it. The subeditor does not 'know' your book in the way that you do and cannot be expected to intuitively grasp what you had in mind when you wrote a sentence or a paragraph if it is unclear.

Remember, too, that this is not the time to rewrite part of your manuscript. All that must have been completed with the final draft. Any rewriting at this stage also means re-editing. The subeditor will have to consider any new material that you have added in the light of what is already in the text and this is bound to slow up the editing process.

If anything remains unclear at this stage, this is your last chance to get things right. In particular, make sure that you answer all the queries relating to *references* appropriately. Again, the subeditor cannot be expected to look up bibliographical references and will expect you to supply full and accurate details if these are missing from your manuscript. Try to deal with the subeditor's queries by return of post.

About this time, too, you are likely to be sent an *author's questionnaire*. This is a form that asks you for details about yourself, your job, your professional life and about the book you have written. You are usually asked to describe the nature of the book in a sentence, in a short paragraph and in some detail. These various descriptions are used by the publishers for different purposes. Some are used to help compose the 'blurb' – the writing on the back cover. Others are used for marketing purposes. You are also asked to help identify the readership for your book and whether or not it would suit particular courses as a textbook. Be accurate and realistic about these issues. It is not appropriate simply to write 'all health-care students on all health-care courses'. Be specific and take the completion of this questionnaire seriously; the publisher does.

Stage 7   The Proofs

Once the completed manuscript has been accepted, you are usually due an advance on royalties which helps to counteract some of the pain of writing. Some publishers pay an advance on the signing of contracts as well as on acceptance of the manuscript but you will have checked this before you signed the contract. Now all you have to do is wait again. This will probably be the longest wait of all. The processing of a book manuscript into a printed book is always a lengthy one. Some publishers have the typesetting and printing done in the Far East which adds even more time to the process. Eventually, though, you will see the pages of the book in proof form. Normally, these days, you can expect to see 'page proofs'. With these, every two pages of the book are printed out onto one larger sheet. You can get a good idea from these what the final book will look like.

Your task at this point is to proof read. It must be emphasized that the aim of proof reading is to find printers' errors and editing errors: it is *not* the time to make textual changes. You cannot rewrite passages of text at this stage. Major (and even minor) changes at this stage are very expensive and if you insist on changes being made you may be expected to pay for them. Check the proofs carefully.

After the proofs have been returned or sometimes at the same time, you may be asked to compile an index. Again, this will depend on your contract. It may also depend on your preference. Some authors prefer to make their own indexes, others are happy to have a trained indexer make them. If you do make your own, work quickly but accurately. Time is important at this stage and the publishers are working to tight time schedules.

Stage 8   The Publication

Then, another wait. This always feels the longest because you have already seen the proofs. Little compares, though, with seeing the final, completed book. Normally, your contract will allow you to claim about six complimentary copies, which may follow after the initial one. Your first copy may also arrive before publication date so don't rush out to the shops to see if it's in. Don't expect, either, that all of the bigger bookshops will automatically stock it. Yours is likely to be a fairly specialized text so it may be stocked by the big, main bookshops and the college and university bookshops but is unlikely to be on sale at airports and railway stations.

Once you have been through these eight stages, you may feel you want a break. Or you may feel that you want to push ahead with another book. If you do, just go back to stage 1 and start again; the process is exactly the same.

REPRINTS AND SECOND EDITIONS

When a book is published, the commissioning editor and their team have to estimate how many copies the book is likely to sell. If these expectations are exceeded, the publishers will probably *reprint* the book. Just before they do this, they may ask if you have spotted any further typographical errors in the book and invite you to rectify these. This is never an invitation to *rewrite* parts of the book. A reprint is nearly always simply a reissue of the book as it stands.

After about four years, if the book is still selling well, the publishers may approach you to consider writing a second (or subsequent) edition. Alternatively, if you know the book is selling well (and you will know this from royalty statements) you may suggest the idea to the publisher.

The preparation of a second or subsequent edition of a book is something of a balancing act. On the one hand, you are given the chance of updating the original book and introducing new material. On the other hand, you are required to maintain the character and (usually) the layout and format of the original text. New editions are often bought by people who bought the first edition of the book. While they want to see changes, they don't usually want to find that you have written a completely different book. As a rule of thumb, it is usual to include about 25% of the manuscript as new material. Also, it is common practice not to change the *title* of the book in any way. Again, people want to know that they are buying a book which is similar to the first edition, even if the contents have been updated.

If a second edition proves popular and it is clear that a third edition is likely to be requested, it makes good sense to begin to collect material for it as you go along. Authors who have written 'classic' texts often make a point of keeping their reference databases up to date at all times and collect new material as part of their everyday work. All of this research makes the writing of a new edition much easier than if you have to start from scratch each time. It is also notable that writing further editions of books is often slightly easier and much more enjoyable than writing the first. The starting point for such an enterprise is a thorough re-reading of the original book. During this process, it is important to mark up the margins of the book to indicate to yourself where changes might be made. Careful reading at this stage will help you to avoid *repeating* yourself at various points in the book – a distinct possibility if you forget that you have written a substantial section on something in Chapter 2, only to return to it in Chapter 5!

WRITER'S BLOCK

This is something that happens to most people who want or have to write. It is the situation in which you find yourself unable to write anything at all. This may be a short-term process or it can last for a considerable time. Clearly, when it does happen, something needs to be done.

About three months before I started preparing the second edition of this book, I suffered from about six weeks of writer's block. Having written more than 20 books and over 200 published papers, I suddenly found myself unable to type more than two or three words without stumbling over them. Given that I work in a university department where the expectation is that I *will* write in various sorts of ways, this was a blow. What I did worked for me: it may or may not work for you.

First, I took this as a sign of burnout, of writing and work-related stress. I made the decision, therefore, to stop writing altogether for at least a month and read only novels during this period. The forced break meant that my anxiety levels were temporarily reduced. When I came back to writing, I used a type of behavioural approach. I limited myself initially to writing a maximum of 500 words an evening, twice a week. Prior to this bout of writer's block, I would often write a few thousand words on a number of occasions during the week. Again, the enforced limitation meant that I was not putting undue pressure on myself to achieve. The other 'rule' was that I would not be too critical of what I had written, that I would allow it to stand as I wrote it. Within two weeks I seemed to be over the block and able to write fairly freely again. One thing I have learned from the episode, though, is not to write too often and for too long.

Other people have recommended other ways of dealing with writer's block. Simply put, these are as follows.

1. Open up a new file on your word processor or start with a fresh piece of paper and put the word 'The' on the top line. This sounds ridiculously simple but it does mean that you have begun to write *something*. You are no longer faced with an empty screen that seems to demand huge numbers of words that you do not have at your disposal. Also, any number of sentences can start with *the* and this makes the process of getting started easier.

2. Make writing a habit. Treat it as just another job that you have to do. Neither decide that you 'enjoy writing' nor that you 'hate writing'. Just write.

3. Do something completely different for a few days. Break your usual routines.

4. Write somewhere different. If you are used to writing in the dining room, move to the bedroom. If you are used to writing at work, take your work home and write there.

5. Practise *free writing*. That means, write anything that comes into your head. Express yourself in a *flow of consciousness*. Make no attempt to censor what you write or tidy up your writing. Often, this sort of writing really does free you up to write something useful. In my experience, too, it often produces work that you can use.

6. Start with a cliché. At the top of your page or on the first line of your word processor, begin a sentence such as 'Health care, as always, is changing rapidly ...'. Just having started to write something can help you to write more. Remember, you can always return and edit out the opening cliché. The point is to get you writing.

Also, treat writing as something that can always be improved. You never did write better than you do now. You are always improving by virtue of having more and more experience of the process. Sometimes writer's block is caused by setting too high an expectation of yourself. Learn to compromise. Learn to accept that the piece you have written *will do*. Finally, learn to listen to other people's advice about your work. Strong (1991) offers the following guidelines about how to get feedback on writing.

1. Read your work aloud twice.
2. Don't 'defend' your work.
3. Take notes on what others tell you.
4. Ask questions to clarify what others say.
5. Thank people for their comments.
6. Never apologize for the piece you're asking someone to read.

Peer review of written work is particularly useful. If you work in a group or in a class, it is often useful if you can compare what you have written and allow others to comment on it. Initially, many people find the idea of this terrifying. In the end, though, other people turn out to be very supportive. After all, their work has either been reviewed by the group or will be reviewed at a later date. Consider, then, either sharing your work by using the above guidelines or at least letting other people see a printed copy of your work.

WRITING FOR PUBLICATION WITH A COMPUTER

The aim here is to identify some of the ways in which using a computer can make a direct difference to the writing of journal papers and books. Whilst not everyone gets used to writing directly with a keyboard, the fact that a paper or a book does not have to be rewritten (by a copy typist) is the overriding advantage of learning to use a computer to communicate your thoughts. If you do decide to invest in and use a computer with a word-processing package, consider the following methods of making the process even easier.

- Work with the line setting set to single spacing, even though your final printout will be double spaced. If you work with single line spacing, you can see more of your work and the eye does not have to move as far to scan the words. Scrolling through documents will be faster, too.
- Consider working with very wide margins, whilst you are typing. This has the effect of making the screen look like this:
  The advantage of this sort of setting is that it allows you to see a lot of your work very easily. You no longer have to scan long sentences but, instead, your work is broken up into small, visible chunks.
- Try to learn all the functions of your word processor. It is surprising how easy life can be once you let the computer do most of the more routine tasks for you.

- If your word processor supports them, make liberal use of macros (the linking of a series of keystrokes to a single keystroke). Well-thought-out macros can save you time when cutting and pasting, spell checking, word counting and backing up your work.
- Count words regularly. Regular word counts improve the style and consistency of your work by ensuring that you stick to the word limits that you set yourself at the proposal stage.
- Put references in at a later date, if recalling them whilst writing is difficult. Simply place the following code into your writing wherever a reference should appear (***). Then, when you have finished the bulk of your writing, have the word processor search for all the codes and insert the appropriate references as you go.
- If your word processor supports them, make good use of style sheets to ensure a uniform look to written work, particularly when you are writing a longer project such as a thesis or book. Style sheets can ensure that all your chapter headings and subheadings are identical in style.
- If you have to print out a very long document on a dot matrix printer, consider printing it in bold and draft quality. This is much quicker than printing in near letter quality and looks almost as good.
- Keep long documents divided into smaller sections by having a separate file for each section. Some word processors allow you to pull a number of files together so that you can view the entire project as a whole.
- Consider laying out all your headings and subheadings for your entire project, before you start to type the body of the text. This will ensure uniformity of layout and you will also be encouraged by the regular appearance of subheadings. This method also aids consistency and helps you avoid repetition.
- Despite all these suggestions, keep your word processing simple. Avoid using fancy fonts and italics. Negroponte (1995) sums up this point well when he writes:

> Too much freedom has also had ill effects on our hard-copy output from laser printers. The ability to change font style and size is a temptation that pollutes many present-day university and business documents, which insensitively mix serif and sans serif type of all kinds and sizes: normal, bold and italic, with and without shadows. It takes some deeper understanding of typography to realize that sticking with a single typeface is usually more appropriate, and to change size very sparingly. Less can be more.

- For work that is to be published, avoid elaborate diagrams, particularly ones that use vertical lines. Whilst your word processor may be able to cope with them, such diagrams are expensive to reproduce in published work. As a rule, make sure that tables use only *horizontal* lines to separate sections and lines of figures. Keep tables as simple as possible. This makes them easier to reproduce and easier to read. Also, complicated diagrams may be confusing rather than clarifying. Imagine, for example, that you produce a diagram which contains blocks of words, linked by lines and arrows. Imagine that the diagram is a 'circular' one that links the various blocks of words to one another, round in a circle. There are many diagrams of this sort in health-care and education books. Why, then, might such diagrams be misleading? First, it might be assumed by the reader that the *length* of the connecting lines is important and significant. Second, what appears to be a 'cycle' may not, in fact, be one. The 'cycle' may be artificially imposed on the words in the diagram. In other words, diagrams which are complicated may *misrepresent* the data involved. As a rule, only use diagrams that you are sure will *simplify the understanding of a series of ideas.*

- Write fast and edit later. One of the main advantages of word processing is the editing facility. This releases you from having to think too hard about spelling and sentence construction in your initial drafts.

- Back up your work as a matter of course. Do not be tempted to trust your hard disk, if you have one. All hard disks fail at some time. If your word processor allows it, set it to do automatic backups while you work. Remember, though, that those backups are lost when you turn off the computer. If you are working on a large and important project, consider having at least two sets of backup disks. Keep one set at home and the other at work. Remember, though, to continue to back up both sets. The alternative to *floppy disk* backups is to use a *tape streamer*, a simple tape machine linked to your computer which backs up everything that is on the hard disk. Also, it is possible and relatively economical to install a second hard disk for backup purposes. Some *portable* hard disks are now produced which enable you to make simple and quick backups and to store the backed up files in another location, away from the computer. It seems likely that it will soon be possible, on a regular and easy basis, to write to CD-ROM disks. Whatever method you choose, backups *must* be made. The ideal, of course, would be a form of storage that is so reliable that no backup system is required. At the moment, though, that seems unlikely for the foreseeable future.

- If you are writing for publication, ask your publisher if you can submit your work on disk. Some journals will accept manuscripts in this format. Most book publishers, though, will want a hard (paper) copy as well as the manuscript on disk. Submitting work on disk can help to speed up the processing time at the publishers. Sometimes, you can submit your work via the Internet, using a file attached to an e-mail message. This is discussed in more detail in Chapter 12. When you do submit your hard copy, do not be tempted to use special, 'heavy' paper, in the mistaken belief that such paper will look more professional. All that is achieved is a heavier parcel to take to the Post Office and a larger document for the publishers to work with. Use standard, photocopier paper.

- Consider using a 'notepad' program (such as *Sidekick*), while you work in your word processor. This allows you to make quick memos to yourself as you type. Otherwise, don't be afraid to leave yourself comments as you go. Again, use the *** symbols to indicate the beginning and end of such memos and later do a search for those symbols. The two sets will tell you where the 'memo' starts and ends.

- Consider running off a copy of larger projects in draft printout mode. You can then use this to read through the entire project and you are free to scribble notes and changes all over it. A manuscript often 'reads' quite differently once it is printed out.
- Do not use headers or footers in your final manuscript. If these identify your name in a paper that is being sent out for 'blind' reviewing, then the editor will have to erase that name on each sheet. If you are submitting a book manuscript, the headers and footers will also have to be erased by a subeditor. Make sure, though, that you *number* every page.
- If you are using an inkjet printer, make sure that you have one or two spare ink cartridges. With some printers, the cartridges only print about 100 pages and with a long book manuscript, you may need two or three cartridges. For some reason, it is easy to forget this and start your printing on a Sunday when the shops are shut. The same applies to laser printer cartridges but here a different problem arises. Because printer cartridges for laser printers last so long, it is easy to forget that you have been using yours for some months. When you come to print out a very long document, you suddenly find that only half the pages have been printed.

THE INTERNET FOR WRITERS

The Internet – a huge, worldwide computer network – is not only useful for finding information on the topic you are writing about. It also contains some useful WorldWide Web pages specifically for writers. These two WWW addressses may be useful to you if you do a lot of writing: ·

- The Writers' Site (set up by the Authors' Licensing and Collecting Society) http:/www.alcs.co.uk
- The Society of Authors http://www.writers.org.uk/society

Like most other WorldWide Web sites, these two pages are hyperlinked to a range of other, related Internet pages.

Overall, the Internet is likely to be a valuable resource for most people who have to write within the health professions. There are plenty of medical and medically related pages, bibliographies, contents pages (and even complete editions) of health care-related pages and very much more. Use one of the searching facilities to enter keywords to start off your enquiry. The only drawback to the Internet (apart from its sometimes being slow) is that you can easily be sidetracked by hypertext links to interesting but only tangentially related topics. It pays to stay focused when you are looking for information on the Internet.

I have written in more detail about writing with computers, and writing in general, in *Writing for Health Professionals* (Burnard, 1996).

SUMMARY

Writing is an important aspect of communication in the health professions. This chapter has explored some of the nuts and bolts of the writing process and examined the stages through which you must go if you are to see your written work in print. Writing for publication can be an enjoyable activity and is a vital one for anyone employed in an academic capacity within the health professions. The chapter closed with suggestions about how to speed up and improve your writing for publication with the aid of a computer.

References

Burnard, P. (1996) *Writing for Health Professionals: A Manual for Writers*, 2nd edn, Chapman & Hall, London.
Negroponte, D. (1995) *Being Digital*, Black Arrow, London.
Strong, W. (1991) *Writing Incisively: Do-it-yourself Prose Surgery*, McGraw-Hill, New York.

Further reading

Turk, C. and Kirkman, J. (1989) *Effective Writing: Improving Scientific, Technical and Business Communication*, 2nd edn, E. & F.N. Spon, London.
Wells, G. (1981) *The Successful Author's Handbook*, Macmillan, London.

2 | Assertiveness skills

AIMS OF THE CHAPTER

In this chapter, the following skills and issues are discussed.

- What is assertiveness?
- Why be assertive?
- Assertiveness skills
- Differences between male and female communication styles

WHAT IS ASSERTIVENESS?

We have noted that both caring and working in organizations take their toll on the individual. Sometimes the person's own needs become subsumed within the demands of the organization or profession. One positive way of coping with stress in organizations and in the caring professions is to become more assertive. Assertiveness is often confused with being aggressive but there are important differences. The assertive person can state clearly and calmly what she wants to say, does not back down in the face of disagreement and is prepared to repeat what she has to say, if necessary. Assertiveness, then, is about thinking clearly, being aware of your needs and being able to use the appropriate behaviours to express those needs to others. At the same time, it carries a covert assumption that the assertive person will also respect the needs of others. For acknowledging our own needs must surely involve an appreciation that other people also have needs of their own.

Woodcock and Francis (1983) identify the following barriers to assertiveness.

1. Lack of practice. You do not test your limits enough and discover whether you can be more assertive.
2. Formative training. Your early training by parents and others diminished your capacity to stand up for yourself.
3. Being unclear. You do not have clear standards and you are unsure of what you want.

4. Fear of hostility. You are afraid of anger or negative responses and you want to be considered reasonable.

5. Undervaluing yourself. You do not feel that you have the right to stand firm and demand correct and fair treatment.

6. Poor presentation. Your self-expression tends to be vague, unimpressive, confusing or emotional.

Given that most health professionals spend much of their time considering the needs of others, it seems likely that many overlook the personal needs identified within Woodcock and Francis' list of barriers to assertiveness. Part of the process of coping with stress is learning to identify and assert personal needs and wants.

A continuum may be drawn that represents behaviour ranging from the submissive to the aggressive, with assertive behaviour being the mid-point on such a continuum (Figure 2.1).

Heron (1986) has argued that when we have to confront another person, we tend to feel anxiety at the prospect. As a result of that anxiety we tend to either 'pussyfoot' (and be submissive) or 'sledgehammer' (and be aggressive). So it is with being assertive. When they are learning how to assert themselves, most people experience anxiety and as a result tend to be either submissive or aggressive. Some handle that anxiety by swinging right the way through the continuum. They start submissively, then develop a sort of confidence and rush into an aggressive attack on the other person. Alternatively, other people deal with their anxiety by starting an encounter very aggressively and quickly back off into submission. The level and calm approach of being assertive takes practice, nerve and confidence.

Submissive Approach (Pussyfooting)	Assertive Approach	Aggressive Approach (Sledgehammering)
The person avoids conflict and confrontation by avoiding the topic in hand.	The person is clear, calm and prepared to repeat what she has to say.	The person is heavy-handed and makes a personal attack of the issue.

Figure 2.1 Three possible approaches to confrontation.

Consider the following examples of Heron's three types.

The Pussyfooting Approach

1. 'There's something I want to talk to you about ... I don't really know how to put this ... whatever you do, don't take offence at what I have to say ...'
2. 'I don't expect you will like this but I think it's better that I say it than keep quiet about it ... on the other hand, perhaps its better to say nothing.'
3. 'I know that you have an awful lot of work and I don't want to add to it. Perhaps I ought to discuss what I have in mind with someone else.'

The Sledgehammer Approach

1. 'What you do annoys me. If you had any feelings at all, you wouldn't get home so late ... but that's typical of you.'
2. 'I give up with you. I bet you don't even know what I'm upset about ...'
3. 'Everybody round here is busy. I don't know why you think you're so special. I want you to take on another caseload.'

The Assertive Approach

1. 'I would prefer it if you could get home a little earlier.'
2. 'I'm feeling angry at the moment and I want to discuss our relationship.'
3. 'I would like you to consider taking on Mrs Jones and her family.'

Notice, too, in your own behaviour and that of others, that *posture* and body language often have much to do with the degree to which a statement is perceived by others as submissive, aggressive or assertive. These types of postures and body statements may be described using Heron's three approaches.

The Pussyfooting Approach

1. Hunched or rounded shoulders
2. Failure to face the other person directly
3. Eye contact averted
4. Nervous smile
5. Fiddling with hands
6. Nervous gestures
7. Voice low pitched and apologetic

The Sledgehammer Approach

1. Hands on hips or arms folded
2. Very direct eye contact
3. Angry expression
4. Loud voice
5. Voice threatening or angry
6. Threatening or provocative hand gestures

The Assertive Approach

1. Face to face with the other person
2. 'Comfortable' eye contact
3. Facial expression that is congruent with what is being said
4. Voice clear and calm

What is notable from these three descriptions is that the pussyfooting and sledgehammer approaches can have *physical* as well as psychological effects. The person who frequently adopts one of these two approaches in her dealings with others will often find that she is both physically and emotionally stressed by the experience. Becoming assertive is a potent method of learning to cope with all aspects of personal stress. It can also help to overcome *organizational* stress in that the assertive person is rather more likely to express her own needs and wants and more likely to be heard.

WHY BE ASSERTIVE?

Examples of how assertiveness can be useful include the following situations.

1. When used to express the idea that a person is being asked to do too much by their employer.
2. When used by a person who has never been able to express her wants and needs in a marriage.
3. When used by the health professional facing bureaucratic processes in trying to get help for her client.
4. In everyday situations in shops, offices, restaurants and other places where a stated service is not actually being given.
5. When used by the health professional who is attempting to modify the organizational structure of her work place.

Arguably, the assertive approach to living is much clearer when it comes to dealing with other human beings. The submissive person often loses friends because they come to be seen as duplicitous, sycophantic or as a 'doormat'. On the other hand, the aggressive person is rarely popular perhaps, simply, because most of us don't particularly like aggression. The assertive person comes to be seen as an 'adult' person who is able to treat other people reasonably and without recourse to either childish or loutish behaviour. Hargie, Saunders and Dickson (1987) summarize the functions of assertiveness when they suggest that the appropriate use of assertive interventions can help an individual to:

1. ensure that their personal rights are not violated;
2. withstand unreasonable requests from others;
3. make reasonable requests of others;
4. deal effectively with unreasonable refusals from others;
5. recognize the personal rights of others;
6. change the behaviour of others towards them;

7.   avoid unnecessary aggressive conflicts;
8.   confidently and openly communicate their position on any issue.

All these functions can enable people to reduce their stress levels in interpersonal communication. Much has been written on the topic of assertiveness and the reader is referred to the recommended reading list at the end of this volume. It is worth noting, too, that assertiveness can help in the fight against what Ellis called the 'twelve irrational beliefs' that many people hold (Ellis, 1970).

1.   One must have complete approval from all significant people.
2.   One must be thoroughly competent and achieving.
3.   Undesired events or consequences are horrible and terrible.
4.   People who behave in ways one does not like are bad and should be blamed.
5.   Emotional misery is externally produced and unchangeable.
6.   One should become upset about things that seem fearful.
7.   It is easier to avoid dealing with life's difficulties than to attempt to resolve them.
8.   The past is an unchangeable determinant of current and future behaviour.
9.   Life should be better than it is and it is terrible if solutions to problems are not found quickly.
10. Inertia can produce happiness.
11. Order and certainty are necessary to feel comfortable, even if only through belief in a higher power or being.
12. One's self-evaluation is dependent upon achievements or approval from others.

Alberti and Emmons (1982) identify four major elements in assertive behaviour.

1.   *Intent*. The assertive person does not intend to be hurtful to others by stating his own needs and wants.
2.   *Behaviour*. Behaviour classified as assertive would be evaluated by an 'objective observer' as honest, direct, expressive and non-destructive of others.
3.   *Effects*. Behaviour classified as assertive has the effect on the other of a direct and non-destructive message by which that person would not be hurt.
4.   *Sociocultural context*. Behaviour classified as assertive is appropriate to the environment and culture in which it is demonstrated and may not necessarily be considered 'assertive' in a different sociocultural environment.

Thus Alberti and Emmons invoke some ethical dimensions to the issue of assertiveness. They are suggesting that, used correctly, assertive behaviour is not intended to hurt the other person, should not be perceived as being hurtful and that assertive behaviour is dependent upon culture and context. They further suggest that assertive behaviour can be broken down into at least the following components.

Eye contact

The assertive person is able to maintain eye contact with another person to an appropriate degree.

Body posture

The degree of assertiveness that we use is illustrated through our posture, the way in which we stand in relation to another person and the degree to which we face the other person squarely and equally.

Distance

There seems to be a relationship between the distance we put between ourselves and another person and the degree of comfort and equality we feel with that person. If we feel overpowered by the other person's presence, we will tend to stand further away from them than we would do if we felt equal to them. Proximity in relation to others is culturally dependent but, in a common-sense way, we can soon establish the degree to which we, as individuals, tend to stand away from others or feel comfortable near to them.

Gestures

Alberti and Emmons suggest that appropriate use of hand and arm gestures can add emphasis, openness and warmth to a message and can thus emphasize the assertive approach. Lack of appropriate hand and arm gestures can suggest lack of self-confidence and lack of spontaneity.

Facial expression/tone of voice

It is important that the assertive person is congruent in their use of facial expression (Bandler and Grinder, 1975). Congruence is said to occur when what a person says is accompanied by an appropriate tone of voice and by appropriate facial expressions. The person who is incongruent may be perceived as unassertive. An example of this is the person who says he is angry but smiles as he says it; the result is a mixed and confusing communication.

Fluency

A person is likely to be perceived as assertive if he is fluent and smooth in his use of his voice. This may mean that those who frequently punctuate their conversation with 'ums' and 'ers' are perceived as less than assertive.

Timing

The assertive person is likely to be able to pay attention to his 'end' of a conversation. He will not excessively interrupt the other person, nor will he be prone to leaving long silences between utterances.

Listening

The assertive person is likely to be a good listener. The person who listens effectively not only has more confidence in his ability to maintain a conversation but also illustrates his interest in the other person. Being assertive should not be confused with being self-centred.

Content

Finally, it is important that what is said is appropriate to the social and cultural situation in which a conversation is taking place. Any English person who has been to America will know about the unnerving silence that is likely to descend on a conversation if he uses words such as 'fag' or 'lavatory' in certain settings! So will the person who uses slang or swear words in inappropriate situations. It is important, in being perceived as assertive, that a person learns to use appropriate words and phrases.

A paradox emerges from all these dimensions of assertive behaviour. The assertive person also has to be genuine in his presentation of self. Now if that person is too busy monitoring his behaviour and verbal performance, he is likely to feel distinctly self-conscious and contrived. It would seem that assertiveness training, like other forms of interpersonal skills training, tends to go through three stages and an understanding of those stages can help to resolve that paradox.

- *Stage 1*   The person is unaware of his behaviour and unaware of the possible changes that he may bring about in order to become more assertive.
- *Stage 2*   The person begins to appreciate the various aspects of assertive behaviour, practises them and temporarily becomes clumsy and self-conscious in their use.
- *Stage 3*   The person incorporates the new behaviours into his personal repertoire of behaviours and 'forgets' them but is perceived as more assertive. The new behaviours have become a 'natural' part of the person.

It is suggested that if behaviour change in interpersonal skills training is to become relatively permanent, the person must learn to live through the rather painful second stage of the above model. Once through it, the new skills become more effective as they are incorporated into that person's everyday presentation of self.

BECOMING ASSERTIVE

In developing assertiveness in others, the trainer is clearly going to have to be able to model assertive behaviour herself. The starting point in this field, then, is personal development if it is required. This can be gained through attendance, initially, at an assertiveness training course and later through undertaking a 'training the trainers' course. An increasing number of colleges and extramural departments of universities offer such courses and they are also often offered as evening courses.

Once the trainer has developed some competence in being assertive, the following stages need to be incorporated in a successful training course for others:

Stage 1

A theory input which explains the nature of assertive behaviour, including its differentiation from submissive and aggressive behaviour.

Stage 2

A discussion of the participant's own assessment of their assertive skills or lack of them. This assessment phase may be enhanced by volunteers role playing typical situations in which they find it difficult to be assertive.

Stage 3

Examples of assertive behaviour which the participants may copy. These may be short video film presentations, demonstrations by the facilitator with another facilitator, demonstrations by the facilitator with a participant in the workshop or demonstrations offered by skilled people invited into the workshop to demonstrate assertive behaviour. The last option is perhaps the least attractive as too good a performance can often lead to group participants feeling deskilled. It is easy for the less confident person to feel 'I could never do that'. For this reason, too, it is important that the facilitator running the workshop does not present herself as being too assertive but allows some 'faults' to appear. A certain amount of lack of skill in the facilitator can be reassuring to course participants.

Stage 4

Selection by participants of situations that they would like to practise in order to become more confident in being assertive. Commonly requested situations, here, may include:

- responding assertively to a colleague;
- dealing with clients more assertively;

- returning faulty goods to shops or returning unsatisfactory food in a restaurant;
- not responding aggressively in a discussion;
- being able to speak in front of a group of people or deliver a short paper.

These situations can then be rehearsed using the slow role play method. At each stage of the role play, the participants are encouraged to reflect on their performances and adopt assertive behaviour if they have slipped into being either aggressive or submissive. Sometimes, this means replaying the role play several times. Another learning aid here is the use of what may be called 'perverse role play'. Here, the situation is played out by the participants as *badly as possible*. In other words, the supposedly assertive person is anything but assertive and the 'client' behaves as badly as possible. It is often out of these perverse situations that new learning about what *could* be done occurs.

Stage 5

Carrying the newly learned skills back into the 'real world'. Sometimes, the very act of having practised being assertive is enough to encourage the person to practise being assertive away from the workshop. More frequently, however, there needs to be a follow-up day or a series of follow-up days in which progress or lack of it is discussed and further reinforcement of effective behaviour is offered.

EFFECTS OF BEING ASSERTIVE

In this section you are invited to decide to what degree you are assertive in your relationships with others. First, consider the following areas and think about the degree to which you deal assertively (or otherwise) with other people.

1. At home
2. At work, with colleagues
3. At work, with clients or patients
4. With friends
5. In shops

Now consider the following questions.

1. Which style of confrontation describes your style best?
   a. Pussyfooting
   b. Sledgehammer
   c. Confronting

2. What (if anything) stops you from being assertive?
   a. Fear of rejection
   b. Feelings of inadequacy
   c. Feelings that other people are more important than you
   d. Fear of reprisal
   e. Other feelings

3.   What do you need to do to become more assertive?

4.   What is likely to happen if you become more assertive?

This last question is an important one. If you are going to become more assertive, other people may perceive you differently for a while. If you have had a tendency to be the 'pussyfooting' type, they are likely to see you as rather more pushy. If you have tended towards the 'sledgehammer' approach, they may see you as rather more subdued. Either way, other people are likely to be rather upset by your new 'presentation of self' and to want the 'old you' back. It is during this period that you need most courage and perseverance. The temptation to slip back to old ways is likely to be strong. If you want to deal with the world more on your own terms and to reduce the stress of always being subservient to the needs of others, such courage and perseverance pay off in the longer term.

MALE AND FEMALE FORMS OF COMMUNICATION

Do men and women communicate differently? If so, can we talk about different *styles* of assertiveness? Are we to assume that the differences between men and women can be accounted for mostly in terms of basic physiology or can we include differences associated with the way in which they communicate with each other? If there are differences, are they 'biological' or are they a product of socialization? Do we learn to be 'male communicators' and 'female communicators'? If there are differences in communication, are there different forms of *assertive* communication? These questions are being addressed more frequently in the linguistics and psychology literature.

Tannen, in an important book about the argument for assuming that there *are* basic male/female communication differences (Tannen, 1990), offers the following vignette which illustrates something of that difference. A couple are driving home one evening. The woman says to the man 'Would you like to stop for a drink?'. The man replies 'No'. The woman feels disgruntled as they drive on and later she talks to the man about her feelings. He is unable to understand her feelings. There are, it may be argued, a number of things going on here. First, the woman approaches the idea of stopping for a drink. The man reads this as being a direct question about whether or not *he* wants to stop. The woman, on the other hand, would prefer it if the man had taken *her* feelings on the matter into account (for she *wanted* to stop for a drink). He might have asked 'What would *you* like to do?'. The woman, as a result, is hurt by the man's response. The man, on the other hand, prefers to think that he was simply answering the question and wished that the woman would say what she meant more directly. According to Tannen, what we are seeing here is two different *styles* of communication. The woman is taking a more 'sociable' position on the issue, while the man is treating it in a more 'businesslike' way.

If there are essential differences between male and female forms of communication, then we would do well to avoid generalizing about assertive communication.

It seems possible that there may be 'male' assertiveness and 'female' assertiveness. To assume that there is one possible pattern for acting assertively may be to gloss over some important issues between the sexes. Tannen (1990) comments as follows:

> The desire to affirm that women are equal has made some scholars reluctant to show they are different, because differences can be used to justify unequal treatment and opportunity. Much as I understand and am in sympathy with those who wish there were no differences between woman and men – only reparable social injustice – my research, others' research and my own and others' experience tell me it simply isn't so. There *are* gender differences in ways of speaking, and we need to identify and understand them. Without such understanding, we are doomed to blame others or ourselves – or the relationship – for the otherwise mystifying and damaging effects of our contrasting conversational styles.

From a simply observational point of view – and one not backed up, as yet, by research – it is possible to suggest the following differences that sometimes occur between male and female forms of communication. You may want to add to the list or to quarrel with it.

- In mixed group discussions, men often try to dominate the discussion or to 'take over' the group.
- Men often want to take a 'straightforward' and apparently 'logical' view in a discussion where women may be less clearcut.
- Men and women often communicate differently from a non-verbal point of view. Consider, for example, how each of the sexes *sits* and uses the space that they occupy.
- Male and female *explanations* of a series of events may well be different, as may be the telling of the story of the events themselves. Events may be construed differently by each sex.

I have found it instructive to compare general communication patterns between my teenage daughter and son and I have heard of similar 'differences' reported by others. After any social event, my daughter will ring various friends and offer detailed accounts of what has happened, including mention of the people who were there, the conversations that were held, what was done and so on. The sequence of events is thus rehearsed in various ways. My son, on the other hand, will often report on a social event simply in terms of 'It was all right' and offer little in the way of detail. Nor will he phone friends to discuss and describe the event. It is as though, for my daughter, a social event is not complete without a detailed recounting of it, preferably to a number of people. Whereas, for my son, once a social event has passed, it is confined to history and not particularly worth describing in detail. This, clearly, is not empirical evidence for the existence of fundamental differences between gender groupings but many people that I have talked to about these issues report similar 'findings'.

These may be contentious issues but they need to be considered in the context of assertiveness. Assertiveness is not simply a set of rules and principles to be learned but is in many ways culture specific and culture determined. There may even be such things as 'female assertiveness' and 'male assertiveness'. We should be careful, though, in taking this point too far for it could be offered as an excuse for men to adopt types of 'male' behaviour that are compromising to women. Nor might we want to adopt an *essentialist* view of all this: that in some way, these behaviours are 'wired in' to male and females. Instead, we might say that boys and girls are socialized in many different ways and that these socialization processes last well into adult life. We would, perhaps, all do well to observe and be sensitive to gender differences in communication and not rush to assume that there has to be a 'common' mode of communication. Tannen (1990) adds a gloss to the point when she writes:

> Sociologist Erving Goffman points out that inequality due to differences in race and ethnicity disappears when people of the same race or ethnic background close the doors to their own homes. But in private, personal places that we cherish as havens from the outside world, inequality based on gender comes into its own. Not only do we not escape such discrimination in our most intimate relationships, but we can hardly conceive of them apart from gender-based alignments that are inherently asymmetrical – implying a difference of status. We cannot take a step without taking stances that are prescribed by society and gender specific. We enact and create our gender, and our inequality, with every move we make.

The question of how people of either gender might change is also fraught. For women, there may the question of how to express the sorts of changes in male behaviour that they would like to see – especially in male partners. Hite (1988) described some of the problems this way:

> Many women know they are not getting equal emotional support, esteem or respect in their relationships. And yet it can be difficult to describe definitively to a man just how he is projecting diminishing attitudes. Some of the ways this happens are so subtle in their expression that, while a woman may wind up feeling frustrated and on the defensive, she can find it almost impossible to say just why: pointing to the subtle things said or done would look petty, like overreacting. But taken all together, it is no surprise when even one of these incidents can set off a major fight – or, more typically, another round of alienation which never gets resolved.

Men may also have difficulty in changing their way of relating to other people. Goldberg (1976), in describing some of the problems of male and female changes, had this to say on the issue:

> The man who in moments of honest reflection asks himself, 'What is in all this for me? What am I getting, and what can I expect in the future?' may

find himself at a considerable loss to answer positively or optimistically. Her changes in combination with his own rigidity have put him up against the wall. If he persists in his old ways, he stands accused of chauvinism and sexism. If he stretches himself to take on new responsibilities without making equal demands and throwing off parts of his traditional harness, he will only find himself overloaded and strained to the breaking-point. If he lets go of the traditional masculine style completely, he may find to his terror that he is becoming invisible, unsexy and unworthy in the eyes of most women and even most other men, who turn away from a man who is without a job, status and power.

We might, of course, take issue with Goldberg in acknowledging that concepts such as 'sexiness' and 'worthiness' *must* be bound up with traditional male roles. We might suggest instead, that *either* concepts such as sexiness and worthiness can be linked just as easily with modified masculine roles *or* that sexiness and worthiness do not have to arise as part of any such debate. There also seems to be an underlying suggestion in Goldberg's commentary that men *could* become as invisible as some women were they to modify their roles and that the whole idea of invisibility is rightly an anathema to them. He seems to ignore the possibility that many women may have felt 'invisible' in this way. We should note, though (and in no sense as an excuse for Goldberg's points), that he was writing 20 years ago and it is to be hoped that many things on the gender front have since been addressed more clearly. But therein lies the difficulty of the gender issue: merely to discuss it is to declare a position. It is impossible for us (because we are of a gender, ourselves) to adopt a truly objective position on the matter. Nor, one suspects, if there are differences between the sexes, are we truly able to empathize with the other's position. This raises the conundrum of whether or not men and women can ever really understand each other fully or whether 'full understanding' can only occur within the sexes (between two women or between two men). But, stated in that way, it may seem unlikely that there is such exclusivity about understanding. Most of us, I suspect, would like to think that, to some degree at least, we understand one or more persons of the opposite sex.

What is notable, perhaps, in both of the quotations above is that the issue of *power* arises in both of them, covertly in the passage about women in which it is noted that women may have to try to *explain* their positions to men and overtly in the passage about men in which some men *acknowledge* the power dynamic. It seems likely that many of the interactions between men and women are concerned with power relationships and, presumably, this is also true within the gender groups.

The other issue that is beyond the remit of this book is the issue of assertiveness and gender differences between the various sexualities (hetero/homo/bi-sexuality). Much of the literature on communication assumes a heterosexist position. If we are not careful, we too get drawn into 'male versus female' roles as if these were the only two sorts. Devor (1989) acknowledges how, traditionally, gender attributions were made.

1. Every individual was assumed to be male or female, with no one 'in between'.
2. The physical characteristics and traits of behaviour of individuals were interpreted as masculine or feminine according to a dominant gender scheme.
3. Gender cues were routinely weighed and assessed, within the confines of permissible gender status behaviour patterns.
4. Gender differences thus constituted and reconstituted were applied back to concretized sexual identities, with 'crossgender' elements filtered out.
5. Actors monitored their own appearance and behaviour in accordance with 'naturally given' sexual identity.

Again, we must be wary of making too many generalizations about people's behaviour based on gender or on stereotypes of gender and of the various sexualities that people have adopted. Health professionals should be particularly sensitive to gender and sexuality difference and yet the health professions provide classic models of gender division: very many doctors are men and very many nurses are women. Perhaps we need to understand the gender and sexuality divisions within our own professions before we attempt to more fully understand those in the worlds of our patients and clients. Or, perhaps, understanding the one will give us insights into the other.

PROBLEMS WITH ASSERTIVENESS

Life is rarely as straightforward as some of the books on assertiveness would have you believe. Sometimes, it is not simply a question of living your life assertively. There are times when it is appropriate to back down, to decide *not* to be assertive. Perhaps the point is to exercise choice in the matter.

The second problem is that we have to decide what counts as assertive behaviour. It is probably impossible to establish some sort of 'assertiveness gold standard'. What counts as assertiveness is a question of value judgement. I might think that I am acting assertively, whilst another might view my actions as aggressive. Assertive *style* is relatively idiosyncratic and personal. Further, it is always occurring in context. Other people are free to make their own judgements about whether or not our behaviour is assertive or otherwise. Again, what I see as a particular type of behaviour may be viewed by others quite differently. This issue is addressed further at the end of Chapter 4. Central to all the debates about communication and about assertive communication is the question of meaning. How do we understand another person's intentions? Are our interpretations of what other people say 'correct'? Is the speaker's intention the only thing to be considered or should we see meaning as contextual and born out of both the speaker's intention and the listener's interpretation?

Finally, assertiveness has a cultural component. Not every culture values assertiveness. Furnham (1979) expressed this clearly as follows:

... the concept of assertiveness is culture bound, and particularly North American. In many other cultures, asserting oneself in the way that is normative in North America and parts of Europe is neither encouraged nor tolerated. Humility, subservience, and tolerance are valued above assertiveness in many cultures, especially for women. Furthermore, the lack of assertiveness is not necessarily a sign of inadequacy or anxiety, though in instances it may be.

This, then, is an early reminder to remember context and cultural difference. Health-care professionals come into contact with people from many different cultures. To assume that everyone will value and appreciate assertive behaviour is to seriously misread crosscultural dialogue. An intriguing question remains, however, about the degree to which all health-care professionals in North American and northern European settings should learn to be assertive *amongst themselves*. Traditionally, for example, the medical profession has tended to dominate the health professions and there are lots of historical and legal reasons why this has been the case. As other professionals become more autonomous and more 'equal' to the medical profession, it might be argued that they should learn assertiveness so as to help establish and maintain this equality. On the other hand, the cultural issue remains an important one. Many health-care professionals will also be from other countries and other cultures. Further, all health-care professionals will be working with patients and clients from other countries and cultures. It remains, therefore, a contentious issue as to whether or not health education curricula should adopt assertiveness as a topic for teaching across the board. Rakos (1991), in a detailed book about the theory, research and training of assertiveness, offers the following view of assertiveness training 'as a fad':

> [assertiveness training] as a fad, however, seems unlikely to survive past the eighties. The reason partly resides in market mechanisms – after all, how many people can enrol in endless 'courses'? However, the integrity of the scientific underpinnings of AT may also have played a role in the depopularization of AT. The early deluge of studies that showed AT effectively taught the basic response components of assertion has been followed by a more sophisticated research that has clearly demonstrated the complexity of assertiveness.

Rakos, then, usefully summarizes some of the problems of taking too simple a view of human communication and highlights the need to be aware of the increasing amount of research being published in the field of communication in general and assertiveness in particular.

SUMMARY

In order to care for others we must become more clear about our own needs and wants. If we want to reduce interpersonal stress we need assertiveness skills. The chapter has covered the nature of assertiveness, raised various questions about the validity and appropriateness of assertiveness and briefly explored the question of male and female forms of communication. It has also identified and discussed some limitations of assertiveness.

References

Alberti, R.E. and Emmons, M.L. (1982) *Your Perfect Right: A Guide to Assertive Living*, Impact, San Luis Obispo, California.

Bandler, R. and Grinder, J. (1975) *The Structure of Magic, Vol I*, Science and Behavior Books, San Francisco, California.

Devor, H. (1989) *Gender Bending: Confronting the Limits of Duality*, Indiana University Press, Bloomingdale.

Ellis, A. (1970) *The Essence of Rational Psychotherapy: A Comprehensive Approach to Treatment*, Institute for Rational Living, New York.

Furnham, A. (1979) Assertiveness in three cultures: multidimensionality and cultural difference. *Journal of Clinical Psychology*, **30**, 429–32.

Goldberg, H. (1976) *The Hazards of Being Male*, Signet, New York.

Hargie, O., Saunders, C. and Dickson, D. (1987) *Social Skills in Interpersonal Communications*, 2nd edn, Croom Helm, London.

Heron, J. (1986) *Six Category Intervention Analysis*, 2nd edn, Human Potential Research Project, University of Surrey, Guildford, Surrey.

Hite, S. (1988) *Women and Love*, Viking, London.

Rakos, R.E. (1991) *Assertive Behaviour: Theory, Research and Training*, Routledge, London.

Tannen, D. (1990) *You Just Don't Understand: Women and Men in Conversation*, Virago, London.

Woodcock, M. and Francis, D. (1983) *The Unblocked Manager: A Practical Guide for Self-Development*, Gower, Aldershot.

3

Self-awareness skills

AIMS OF THE CHAPTER

In this chapter, the following issues and skills are discussed.

- The nature of self-awareness
- Self-awareness skills
- Self-presentation

WHAT IS SELF-AWARENESS?

The argument is often forwarded that we need to know something about ourselves in order to help others. The point is a contentious one: there is, as yet, little empirical evidence to support the notion that 'self-awareness' necessarily makes for a better practitioner. In a common-sense sort of way, though, it would seem reasonable to assume that if we are to be *seen* as caring and sensitive in our practice, then we need to be able to *notice* what it is we do. We need, in other words, to become *reflexive*. This chapter explores some ideas about self-awareness and also notes some difficulties with the concept.

The point may be raised, at once, whether it is reasonable to talk about self-awareness *skills*. This is a difficult issue. Is self-awareness something that involves skills or is it an attitude, a frame of mind, a disposition? The term 'self-awareness skills' is used guardedly, then, in this chapter in the realization that it is not perfect but in the absence of other, more suitable words.

PHILOSOPHERS AND THE SELF

Talking of 'the self' is no easy task. If we are not careful, we get caught up with ideas that our 'self' somehow exists separately from the rest of us. Or that 'selves' are separate in some way from 'bodies'.

The notion of 'self' is closely tied up with that of *identity* – who we and others think we are and how we see ourselves. This identity includes a sense of being separate from others (on one level), being similar to others (on another) and being much the same as others (on yet another level). It also involves constructs such as confidence, esteem – or lack of it – sexuality and sexual identity and so on.

The existential school of philosophy discussed the issue under the heading of 'ontology': the study of being. To talk of the self was to talk of something more than just bodily existence. It was to describe the fact of being a conscious, knowing human being rather than simply an object. For the existentialists, as for other philosophers, what marked out persons as different from other objects in the world was *consciousness* – the fact that we are able to *reflect* on our being-in-the-world. We 'know we are here', whereas we can imagine that other objects such as furniture or plants have no such reflexive ability. Whilst we may like to think that the cat sitting in front of the fire 'knows' that it is in the world, we have little evidence, as yet, on whether or not this is the case.

Sartre (1956) wrote of 'authenticity', the state of true and honest presentation of being. The authentic person, for Sartre, was one who consistently acted in accordance with her own values, wishes and feelings, making no attempt to adopt a facade. That person also recognized the 'being' of others and realized that when she was with someone else, that other person was also a conscious, valuing, thinking being. For if we can identify our own situation in the world as conscious, valuing and thinking, we must, by extension, realize that all other people are in the same position. To identify our own position in the world is also to acknowledge everyone else's. If we are human, so must all other people be. This, then, is not just a normative position but also an *ethical* one. For, if we acknowledge our own humanity, we must acknowledge that of other people. We must act, perhaps, as though other people were like us in our humanity.

Sartre argued that what marked out the human being from other objects in the world was the fact that *existence* comes before *essence*. People first of all exist – there is no 'blueprint' for them – discover themselves as they grow up and make sense of themselves later. They become, as it were, what they make of themselves. There is no plan behind the fact of human existence. Each of us 'invents' himself: we become what we decide we will become. Faced with this responsibility, we are also faced with the realization that, if it applies to us, then it applies to all other people too. If I choose a course of action, then I am sanctioning that course of action: I am deeming it to be a 'right' course of action. By extension, I am also deeming it to be 'right' for others. Thus, when I choose, I choose not only for myself but for all other people too. It is here that Sartre acknowledges the link between subjective human choice and the fact that we live surrounded by other human beings. We neither exist in isolation nor choose in isolation. That we must choose seems to be a fact of life but there is anguish in choosing. For in choosing we always run the risk of limiting other people's choices through our actions. For Sartre, then, it was important that we choose ourselves 'knowingly' and in good faith. We must choose carefully but with the full knowledge that we can never know, beforehand, the outcome of those choices. We choose, in a sense, blind. In deciding on our identity, we do so in the certain knowledge that we do not know how things will turn out. And this is perhaps the paradox. In choosing ourselves, we also take a leap in the dark. We choose ourselves without any prior knowledge of what we are going to be like as a result of such choosing. We also need to take account of other people's ability to choose. They too are busy defining themselves and we must bear in mind the fact of other people's ability to choose as we 'invent' ourselves.

Sartre acknowledged, too, that with freedom comes full responsibility. One cannot be 'free' and yet 'not responsible'. For example, it would be impossible for me to say: 'I am free to do as I choose as long as I ask my wife, first'. If I am free, then only I can be responsible for what I do.

Martin Buber (1958) referred to the I–Thou relationship, the meeting of two people who respect each other's humanity. He contrasts the I–Thou relationship with the I–It relationship. The person who adopts an I–It stance in relationship with another person does not recognize the other as a human being (with all that involves) but treats the other as an 'object'. There are plenty of examples of health-care professionals turning other people into objects. We do this when we refer to people by their medical labels. We do it when we refer to someone as an 'appendix' or a 'schizophrenic'. They have stopped being living, breathing human subjects similar to ourselves, and become 'things'. On the other hand, we might argue that some objectification of this sort is inevitable. If we always stopped to think of the humanity of the other person, we might be unable to carry out some of the tasks that are asked of us as health professionals. Indeed, it might be argued that the I–Thou relationship is at the core of the health-care relationship. Without the recognition of the 'person' in front of us, we cannot really be said to be engaging fully with that person.

The notion of the I–Thou relationship, however, applies as much to relationships between health professionals as between professionals and their clients or patients. Some senior health professionals can tend to treat more junior ones as 'objects'. There are examples, for instance, of senior medical staff talking to medical students as if they were somehow of a different order or class. The same hierarchical set of relationships can be seen in the nursing profession when senior nurses address very junior ones in dismissive ways. One of Buber's points was that to be consistently human, we must always respect the humanity of the other person and hold the other person in an I–Thou relationship. It should in theory be easier to treat colleagues in this way for, after all, colleagues are not generally expressing the pain that might be expressed by clients or patients. However, intercolleague relationships also involve *power* and power relationships are often more successfully played out if the one who holds the power can treat the one who does not as an 'object'. If the I–Thou relationship is evident at all times, then the power dynamic may not be so easy to administer. Perhaps as we see less overt power being exercised by health professionals – at least in the therapeutic arena – we will see more of a uniform development of the I–Thou relationship.

R.D. Laing wrote of the 'true' and 'false' self (Laing, 1959). The true self, according to Laing, is the inner, private sense of self. The false self is the outer, often pretending sense of self. Laing suggested that the true self often watches what the false self is doing and a sense of contempt is experienced. The false self is often compliant to the demands of others and can be artificial and insincere. In Sartre's terms, the false self acts inauthentically.

The person who has a strong sense of the true self, who is able to act authentically and genuinely is deemed by Laing to have ontological security: security and strength of being. Such security can make the person feel able to act rather than feel acted upon, to make decisions and to feel generally more autonomous. Such a person is also likely to respect the autonomy and self-respect of others. This is not to be confused with selfishness or arrogance – quite the opposite. The ontologically secure person is all too aware of human frailty but, despite it, remains determined to act in a genuine and honest way. It takes courage to be this way. On the other hand, it is difficult to sustain an argument for Laing having identified a 'true' self in this way. Why should we assume that any particular presentation of self is more 'true' than any other? We might instead argue that we have *different* presentations of self in differing situations. We are sometimes this way and sometimes that: our personalities may be more plastic and less well formed than we would sometimes like to think. Also, there are numerous external factors that come into play and which impinge on our sense of self. We are more comfortable and confident with some people than with others. We can more confidently speak of 'being ourselves' with some people than with others. But these may simply be figures of speech. Instead, we might argue that we offer different facets of ourselves in different social situations.

We might even go as far as to say that we simply 'make ourselves up', that there is no consistent self and that the only truth is that we are in a constant state of flux. Clearly this is literally true of our physical selves: our cells are dying and some are regenerating all of the time. By extension, it may be argued that the same is true of our 'sense of self'. Because this is a difficult idea to live with, we choose to imagine that we have a far more consistent sense of self than is actually the case. From Sartre's point of view, perhaps, we would not simply be authors of our own existence but also continuous writers of it. There is, of course, a major objection to be stated about this point of view: if we *do* continuously 'make ourselves up', how is it that others recognize us and we them?

We can see examples of Sartre's and Laing's ideas in health-care practice. When I was a patient in hospital, I became very aware of how some health-care professionals adopt the 'role of the health-care professional' as they enter a ward: they suddenly become 'someone else'. It is as though they leave part of themselves behind as they go to work. They have one 'self' for their patients and another for friends and colleagues. If we notice that we are 'acting the role of the health-care professional' in talking with patients, rather than being ourselves, then we are acting in an inauthentic manner. On the other hand, the point is a moot one. In the end, who is to say that the 'professional' self is any more or less 'me' than the 'real self'? The only way of answering this is to say that we know when we are 'putting on a front'. Similarly, we know when we are simply 'being ourselves'.

The health-care professional who begins to develop self-awareness can, perhaps, monitor her behaviour and note tendencies towards adopting such a veneer. On the other hand, the development of such a veneer might, in many ways, be a coping mechanism to help us to deal with situations that would otherwise be unbearable. We should not always assume that coping mechanisms are somehow a sign of weakness. The fact is that we have to cope and in the health professions we are often called upon to cope with situations that are taxing and difficult. They are often situations which others choose not to cope with. Sometimes, then, we need to develop a different facet of self – a *coping* facet.

The existential view of self was most clearly defined by Carl Rogers, father of the client-centred approach to counselling and of student-centred learning. It is worth quoting Rogers at some length here, as the following passage sums up many of the points identified in the discussion above and is one of Rogers' clearest statements of his philosophical position regarding the concept of self. Further, the statement also indicates where Rogers stood in relation to the psychodynamic approach of Freud and the behavioural position of Skinner:

> For the behaviourist, man is a machine, a complicated but nonetheless understandable machine, which we can learn to manipulate with greater and greater skills until he thinks the thoughts, moves in the directions and behaves in the ways elected for him. For the Freudian, man is an irrational being, irrevocably in the grip of his past and of the product of that past, his unconscious.
>
> It is not necessary to deny that there is truth in each of these formulations in order to recognize that there is another perspective. From the existential perspective, from within the phenomenological internal frame of reference, man does not simply have the characteristics of a machine, he is not simply a being in the grip of unconscious motives: he is a person in the process of creating himself, a person who creates meaning in life, a person who embodies a dimension of subjective freedom. He is a figure who, though he may be alone in a vastly complex universe and its destiny, is also able in his inner life to transcend the material universe; he is able to live dimensions of his life which are not fully or adequately contained in a description of his conditionings or of his unconscious.

(Rogers 1967)

We may, of course, take issue with Rogers' insistence that a person is able to 'transcend the material universe', for to do so might be to suggest that we can comprehend that universe. Rogers also seems to want to satisfy everyone with his appeal to the occasional appropriateness of the Skinnerian or Freudian approaches. In a sense, the existential approach must be 'all or nothing'. You cannot, on the one hand, argue for individual freedom and personal authorship of self and on the other suggest that Skinner and Freud could be incorporated into such a possible world. But Rogers 'does not deny the truth' of those Skinnerian and Freudian formulations. What Rogers has done, however, is to free people from the idea that we are either necessarily products of our past *or* simply machines to be manipulated. Instead, Rogers argues, we are each in our own driving seat. We are, as Sartre suggests, creating ourselves.

OTHER APPROACHES TO THE SELF

Psychologists have approached the concept of self from a variety of points of view. Some have attempted to analyse the factors that go to make up the self rather in the way that a cook might try to discover the ingredients that have gone into a cake. Others have argued that there are certain consistent aspects of the self that determine to some extent the way in which we conduct our lives.

Psychoanalytical theory, for instance, argues that early childhood experiences profoundly affect and shape the self, determining how, as adults, we react to the world about us. Childhood experiences, in this model, lay foundations of the self which may be modified through the process of growing up but which nevertheless stay with us throughout our lives. Such view is 'deterministic': our present sense of self is *determined* by earlier life experiences. The formation of self, for the psychoanalysts, can be traced back to childhood. 'Self' is something that develops gradually out of our experiences of life and other people – particularly, perhaps, early experiences. For the psychoanalysts, too, problems of self in later life can be traced directly back to early experiences. The problem, it seems to me, is in being sure that such links exist. In the end, it seems unlikely that we can ever demonstrate, conclusively, that any adult presentation of self was necessarily *caused* by earlier events and experiences.

Other psychologists acknowledge problems with reductionist theories – theories that attempt to analyse the self into parts. They prefer to view the self from a holistic or Gestalt perspective. The Gestalt approach argues that the totality of the self is always something different from and larger than the sum of the aspects that make it up. Just as we cannot discover the true nature of a piece of music by examining the piece note by note, neither can we understand the self, completely, by analysing it into separate aspects.

Still other psychologists take the view that the sense of self is dynamic and ever changing. There is no core or 'real' self. What we call 'self' at any given time is that moment's set of beliefs, values and ideas that colour our view of the world. George Kelly (1955) suggested the metaphor of 'goggles': we all look at the world, at ourselves and at others, through different goggles that are coloured by our beliefs, values and experiences up to that moment. As our beliefs, values and experiences change, so do the tints of our 'goggles'.

Thus, for Kelly, the person is in a constant state of flux – developing, growing and changing as she encounters life. For Kelly, we *are* what we perceive ourselves to be. Kelly also noted that we are what *other people* perceive us to be, as well. We do not exist in isolation. What we are and who we are depend upon the other people with whom we live, work and relate. Our sense of self often depends upon the reports about us that we receive from others. In this sense, other people are telling us who we are. Also, we may be 'different people' in different situations. The term 'subpersonalities' is sometimes used to acknowledge this idea. Consider, for example, yourself as you are with a good friend, then consider yourself at work, then think about yourself in a social situation in which you don't know very many people. You may find that you present very different aspects of self in the three situations.

As health-care professionals we rely on patients, colleagues, educators and managers offering us both positive and negative feedback. We absorb such feedback and incorporate the bits that we need to into our sense of self. Sometimes reports from others seem important, at other times they seem less necessary.

ASPECTS OF THE SELF

The self is a complicated concept. It is worth emphasizing the word *concept*. The self is not a *thing* in the way that our livers or lungs are 'things'. The notion of self is an abstraction, a way of talking. It is a shorthand for that part of us concerned with thinking, feeling, valuing, evaluating and so forth. Whilst in one sense the mind and body are one, in another they are different, if only in that the body is a *thing*, an object in the world, whilst the mind is a construct. To talk about the 'mind and body' is tricky for it suggests that two similar sorts of items are under discussion. One way of clarifying what is contained within the concept of self is to consider the notion of *personhood*.

If we can identify those basic criteria that distinguish persons from other sorts of things we may be clearer about what it means to talk about the self. Bannister and Fransella (1986) maintain that such a list of criteria for personhood will include at least the following items. It is argued that you consider yourself a person in that you:

- entertain a notion of your own separateness from others: you rely on the privacy of your own consciousness;
- entertain a notion of the integrity or completeness of your experience, so that all parts of it are relatable because you are the experiencer;
- entertain a notion of your own continuity over time: you possess your own biography and live in relation to it;
- entertain a notion of the causality of your actions: you have purposes, you intend, you accept a partial responsibility for the effects of what you do;
- entertain a notion of other persons by analogy with yourself: you assume a comparability of subjective experience.

These criteria bring together many of the ideas discussed above. They acknowledge the person's uniqueness and difference from others; they acknowledge the person's continuity with the past and they acknowledge her relatedness with other people. We do not exist in isolation; we can assume that we share the planet with other people who are, to a greater or lesser degree, like us.

Another way of considering the concept of self is to consider *aspects* of it. Whilst, as we have noted, all the aspects tend to work together in harmony, they are most easily discussed as parts. John Rowan has taken something of a similar approach in his discussion of 'subpersonalities' (Rowan, 1989) which he describes as semi-permanent, semi-autonomous regions of the personality. The analysis offered here is a means of highlighting the complex and multifaceted nature of the concept of self (as we noted above, what individuals call 'self' will vary from person to person). The aspects of self discussed here are:

1. the physical aspect;
2. the spiritual aspect;
3. the darker aspect;
4. the social aspect;
5. the private aspect;
6. the sexual aspect.

It is acknowledged that this is hardly an exhaustive list: we could add to it. But it offers us a starting point for discussing various aspects of self.

THE PHYSICAL ASPECT OF SELF

The physical aspect of the self is the bodily, 'felt' sense of self: it includes the totality of our physical bodies. One way of considering the self, in fact, is to consider that self as being a product of the body: bodies generate 'selves'. After all, the chemistry that goes to make up our bodies is also the chemistry that produces our 'mind' that, in turn, produces our sense of self. The physical aspect of self covers how we feel about our bodies, our sense of body image, our appreciation of how fat or thin we are and so on. It is notable (rather painfully, sometimes) that our own perception of our body is not necessarily the perception that others have. It is notable, from various pieces of research into the topic, that many people have considerably distorted views of their physical selves.

No doubt this is influenced to a greater or lesser degree by the views of the body advanced in magazines and the media. We do compare ourselves with such images and decide, to a greater or less extent, the degree to which we do or do not 'match' the current, popular images of the body. It is notable, too, that those images change considerably over time. In the 1960s, for example, one of the most frequently portrayed images was a 'unisex' one in which male and female body shapes blended to a certain degree. In the 1980s and 1990s, these images changed again, to very definite 'male' and 'female' images. In the late 1990s, we may be seeing another 'blurring of the edges' but driven by a different motive – the ambiguity of hetero- and homosexual positions – a point discussed in more detail below.

THE SPIRITUAL ASPECT OF SELF

Human beings seem to have an inbuilt need to invest what they do with meaning. The spiritual dimension of the person may best be described as that part that is concerned with the generation of meaning. For some, that sense of meaning will be framed in religious terms. For others, meaning may be discovered through philosophy, politics, psychology, sociology and so on. People's meaning systems vary both in their overall structure and in their content.

One thing seems certain: it is meaning (or the search for it) that motivates us for much of the time. Jung (1978) described this quest for meaning as 'individuation': the search for the self which was both lonely and difficult. He suggested that one possible outcome of individuation was the realization of both the individual nature of the person and also the person's unity with all other persons. In this context, Carl Rogers noted that 'what is most personal is most general' (Rogers, 1967): there is a certain universality about the business of being human.

Nor is the spiritual self necessarily linked with religion although, clearly, it may be. Although we acknowledge that the spiritual is to do with a search for meaning, we see that people choose to search for that meaning in very many ways. We may note, for example, in the health professions that those concerned with mental health and social problems are often keen to *interpret* what they find and see. Thus, there are all sorts of theories about how the 'mind' works, what 'happens' when people become mentally ill and so on. It has often been claimed that psychiatrists have taken over as secular priests. They are able to offer 'theories' of what is happening in a situation which appears to be out of control. This sort of 'meaning', in turn, is handed down to nurses, social workers and psychotherapists who adopt the various theoretical positions to 'explain' what it is they are encountering. This, perhaps, is an attempt to *know* something of the spiritual side of other people.

THE DARKER ASPECT OF SELF

There is an aspect in all of us that tends towards the negative. Whilst it has become popular to discuss the positive aspects of the self and to theorize about Maslow's (1972) notion of self-actualization – the realization of our full potential – there seems little doubt that we also have a darker side. Jung described this darker side as the Shadow and wrote about it thus:

> Unfortunately there is no doubt that man is, as a whole, less good than he imagines himself or wants to be. Everyone carries a shadow, and the less it is embodied in the individual's conscious life, the blacker and denser it is ...
>
> (Jung, 1938)

Jung suggests that if we want to become truly self-aware, we must be prepared to explore that darker side to our personalities. No easy task! Most of us would rather deny that side of ourselves or rationalize our negative thoughts and behaviour.

Sometimes, however, we give ourselves away, particularly through the use of the mental mechanism known as 'projection'. With projection, we label others with qualities that are our own but of which we are unaware. Often we notice the bad bits of other people whilst studiously avoiding our own bad bits. This is very evident when we begin to get judgemental and pious about other people. Whilst the Shadow may not be the easiest aspect of ourselves to face, it is likely that acknowledging the darker side can help us to accept the darker side of others.

Perhaps the problem with identifying a darker side to the self is the fact that it assumes a moral dimension. Clearly, that which is identified as darker is, presumably, also identified as 'wrong' or even 'bad'. There are various ways in which we internalize notions of good and bad: through socialization as children, through adherence to a particular religious code, through listening to conscience, by considering what the world would be like if everyone acted as we wish to do.

THE SOCIAL ASPECT OF SELF

The social self is that aspect of the person which is shared with others. It is our presentation of self in various social situations. Consider, for example, yourself at work. Then think of yourself at home. Finally, consider yourself with your closest friend. You may well find that you are thinking of three almost different people! We tend to modify aspects of our presentation of self according to the people we are with and what we anticipate will be their expectations of us.

This social self, then, is closely linked to the self-as-defined-by-others. We do not live as isolated beings. We are dependent upon others to tell us about ourselves. More than that, we *are* different for other people. Consider how the following people view you: your mother, your teacher, your boy or girl friend. In each case, those people will see a different 'you' and yet they are all looking at the same person.

THE PRIVATE ASPECT OF SELF

The private aspect of self is the part that we show only to a few close friends, if we show it at all. It is the part of us that we are caught up in when we are on our own. Think, for example, of the times that you have been at home on your own. At that time, you were likely to be most completely 'yourself': you didn't have to put up any sort of 'front' for others. Instead, you thought and behaved in a rather different way from how you behaved when other people were about. As we get to know other people well, we let them glimpse little bits of the private aspect though it is likely that we reserve some aspects of the private self completely to ourselves.

These aspects of self are just that – aspects. Taken on their own, they do not convey the richness that makes us a human being. That richness is only apparent when all the aspects are working together (and sometimes are in conflict). It is this

Gestalt or whole that makes up the totality of self. Any attempt to break down the self into parts is bound to fail to some degree. We do not operate as 'parts' but as an integrated whole.

THE SEXUAL SELF

Another facet of the self is sexuality. First, there is our general orientation. We may be heterosexual, homosexual or bisexual. It is easy for people of each of these orientations to argue that their own particular one is 'natural', as if there are 'natural' and 'unnatural' orientations. Another view would be that these orientations are simply different. Some, indeed, would claim that bisexuality is the most natural state of affairs and that everyone has elements of both hetero- and homosexuality within them. Otherwise (so the argument goes) we would not have close relationships with people of the same sex at all. Statistically, however, it seems more likely that people 'decide', one way or another, whether they are hetero- or homosexual. The point is to recognize our own sexual orientation and accept it. This may or may not be an easy thing to do and some commentators have even argued that it is possible to choose one's sexual orientation. Arguments also rage as to whether a person's sexual orientation is 'inborn' (what is known as an *essentialist* argument) or whether we are socialized into our sexual orientation. The evidence seems to be that people can remember having a particular orientation from a very early age.

Some writers have argued that many people's sexuality is multifaceted and that it is more accurate to talk of a person's 'sexualities'. This suggests that sexuality is not a single, once and for all thing but that we are all capable of different sorts of sexual experience in different contexts.

The idea of a sexual self goes far beyond the question of physiological differences or even of preferences. Sexual identity is dependent to a considerable degree on relationships and on context. Also, like so many other aspects of self, it depends on the way in which other people see us and relate to us. Consider the following example. Two male patients of the same age are in adjacent hospital beds. The ward is staffed by a number of male and female nurses. One of the men identifies himself as heterosexual, the other as homosexual. Although both have the same *physiological* sense of self, the way in which they perceive themselves and their 'lifeworlds' is likely to be very different. Further, the way in which they perceive *each other* – if each knows the other's orientation – is likely to be different. So is the way in which the various male and female nurses relate to them, based to some degree (but not exclusively) on the nurses' sexual orientation. It has to be said that in the health professions, the orientation of the *helper* or *carer* is often left out of any discussion of patient sexuality.

For the bisexual patient, the sexual sense of self is even more complicated. Generally, bisexuals are 'anonymous' in any given culture. They are often believed to be either (a) sexually promiscuous or having an uncontrollable libido or (b) refusing to acknowledge their 'true' sexual identity. For this and other reasons, the bisexual may often have to choose to 'pass' as either hetero- or homosexual. Also, there are no 'signs' – verbal or otherwise – that enable bisexual people to identify themselves as such to other people. In this sense, the bisexual person can feel something of an outsider. This, in turn, can have an effect on that person's more general sense of self.

The whole issue of the sexual self is given little attention in the literature on health care except when addressing *patients'* sexuality. If we accept the idea that sexuality for everyone is *contextual*, then we see that the sexual self enters into many aspects of the health-care professional/patient relationship. Traditionally, many health-care workers have coped with the issue of undertaking intimate procedures for patients by 'desexualizing' the patient. Doctors and nurses, for example, who have to examine patients' genitals will tend to objectify those patients. This allows both the health-care professional and the patient to act as if the parts of the body in question had no sexual associations. It is as if both parties have instantly denied the sexual issue. Now while health-care professionals may be able to achieve this degree of detachment, the degree to which patients can achieve it is rarely addressed. In other words, we may, as health-care professionals, be fairly comfortable in performing intimate procedures on patients but we cannot assume, nor easily talk about, the degree to which patients can or cannot 'turn off' in this way. It is, of course, essential that health-care professionals can turn off in this way. If they did not, they would presumably find it impossible to attend to patients on intimate issues and presumably patients would find undergoing such examinations impossible. What is in question here is the degree to which either health-care professionals or patients ever get to *talk* about the sexual or non-sexual nature of certain procedures and their respective feelings about them. In a book about communicating with patients, Myerscough (1989) outlines what might be considered the standard way of 'dealing' with the issue of intimate contact and sexuality:

> … doctors require a protective mechanism to professionalize the intimacy that is inseparable from clinical examination, and that they may achieve this only by virtually excluding the patient's sexuality from thought or discussion and by eliminating warmth within the professional relationship.

Whether or not this really is facing the issue or merely skirting around it is open to question. Myerscough makes an even more contentious point when he compares working with children and working with adults:

> A paediatric textbook will describe clearly how to obtain the maximum information from abdominal palpation of children. The basics are to keep smiling in a friendly way, to engage in reassuring, distracting conversation, and to touch with great gentleness, keeping hands in gliding contact with the skin. That sounds perfectly straightforward with a child, but with an adult of the opposite sex, might it not have the overtones of a caress?

Myerscough does not question whether or not the *child* may perceive such behaviour as a 'caress'. Also, he takes a heterosexist position on the issue of the adult's response. Further, he does not question any of the possible feelings that the *doctor* may have. Myerscough seems to assume that the doctor can somehow rise above any sexual feelings that he might have. Now, clearly, it is important that any health professional must be able to do this. To do otherwise would be unethical. However, we need to acknowledge the possibility of the *thought* of a sexual nature occurring.

From the point of view of communication in health care, it would seem that we have a long way to go before we develop the language with which we can talk easily about sexual relationships between health-care professionals and patients. Although this is a contentious area, it may be worth noting that there must be occasions on which health-care professionals 'flirt' with patients (and vice versa). There must also be occasions on which health-care professionals are attracted to their patients (and vice versa). And yet very rarely are these issues addressed either in the literature or, more importantly, in the training and education of health care professionals.

However, indications are that the situation regarding sexuality is changing. Simpson (1996) makes the following observations of the mid-1990s:

> It's a queer old world and getting jolly queerer all the time. Instead of cosmetic tips and boy-meets-girl storylines, something called 'lesbian chic' is used to promote women's magazines and soap operas. Instead of practicing their karate, Hollywood male box-office paramours and action heroes scratch each other's eyes out to play bisexual bloodsuckers and screaming drag queens. ... Instead of offering teen girls real men to lust after, pop music parades hairless boy-bands with unbroken voices in leather chaps and nipple rings. Any red-blooded heterosexualist would be forgiven for thinking the world has turned upside down, as cross-dressing and cross-over turns inversion into the (disorder) of the day in the giddy, topsy-turvy and not a little pervy Nineties.

Even though Simpson is writing ironically and with tongue in cheek when he describes the 1990s as 'pervy', we as health professionals in the 1990s would do well to face a little more squarely some of the facets of communication that are of a potentially sexual nature. We will only do this when we come to terms with sexuality as being much more than biologically or gender based and when we view it as part of the culture and as *contextual*.

MODELS OF THE SELF

What is required now is a model that helps to bring all of these aspects into perspective. In its simplest form, the self as a totality can be seen as being made up of three areas or focuses of interest: thoughts, feelings and behaviour. Each is intimately linked with the other. Thoughts include the processes of ideas, puzzlement and problem solving that make up our mental life. By feelings is meant the emotional aspects of our being: happiness, grief, love, anger, joy, etc. Behaviour refers to any action that we carry out, to the spoken word and to what is usually called non-verbal behaviour: eye contact, facial expressions, gestures, proximity to others.

All three aspects of self, in this simple model, overlap. We cannot think without in some way feeling. Feelings lead to changes in behaviour even though these are sometimes very small changes. Try this. If someone is in the room with you now, just notice them and observe how you can tell that they are thinking or feeling. You will observe changes in eye contact, facial expression or perhaps arm or leg movements. That behaviour changes again if they notice that you are looking at them; their thinking and feeling change as they become aware of you and their behaviour changes as a result. We cannot *stop* behaving any more than we can *stop* communicating.

This interrelatedness of thinking, feeling and behaviour is noticeable from any other starting point. If we ponder for a moment on how we are feeling, such pondering involves thinking and, in turn, a change in behaviour. Here, then, is a starting point for approaching the study of the self. We may study each of the domains and come to know something more about ourselves. As we study each domain and appreciate the connections between all three we gradually peel back the layers to a deeper understanding of who we are.

This is a simple model of the self. A more complex model which, whilst compatible with the first, opens up the domains and expands them is shown in Figure 3.1. It incorporates Jung's work on the four functions of the mind – thinking, feeling, sensing and intuiting (Jung 1978) – and also an adaptation of Laing's concept of the real and false self, alluded to above. It also assimilates some of the aspects of self referred to in the discussion so far.

OUTER SELF	INNER SELF
'Public self'	'Private self'
	Thoughts
Body and behaviour	Feelings
	Senses
	Intuitions

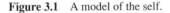

Figure 3.1 A model of the self.

The model is divided into two parts. The outer, public aspect of the self is what others see of us. The inner, private aspect is what goes on in our heads and bodies. In one way, the outer experience is what other people are most familiar with. We communicate the inner experience through the outer. Our thoughts and feelings are all communicated through this outer presentation of self. Of what does it consist?

THE OUTER EXPERIENCE OF THE SELF

At the most obvious, behaviour consists of body movements: the turning of the head, the crossing of arms and legs, walking and running and so on. At a more subtle level the issue becomes more involved. There is a whole variety of less obvious behaviours that convey something about the inner sense of self.

First, speech. Clearly what we say, the words and phrases we use, are a potent means by which we convey thoughts and feelings to others. How we come to choose particular words and phrases, however, depends on our past experiences, our education, our social position, our attitudes, values and beliefs and on the company that we are in when we use those words. Running alongside speech are the non-linguistic aspects of speech: timing, pacing, volume, minimal prompts ('mm' and 'yes'), the use of silence and so on. The use of such non-linguistic aspects can be a powerful way of conveying our inner selves to others. As we noted above, we are always communicating, even when we think we are not!

When we talk to others we invariably look at them. As Heron (1970) notes there can be a wide variety in the intensity, amount and quality of eye contact. When we are embarrassed or upset, for example, we make less eye contact. When we are emotionally close to another person, our eye contact is often sustained. We can learn to become conscious of our use of this most powerful aspect of communication and to monitor the amount and quality of our eye contact. We should also remain aware of the *cultural* differences involved here. People from cultures very different to our own use eye contact in other ways. It is important that we do not interpret such different use of eye contact inappropriately.

Touch is another important aspect of our outer experience. Typically, in this culture, we touch more those people to whom we are close: members of the family, lovers and very close friends. Health care involves a high degree of this personal aspect of human interaction and it is important that, as with eye contact, we learn to monitor and consciously use the facility of touch. It is worth noting, too, that some people are 'high touchers' and others 'low touchers'. Some people like being touched and like touching others while other people are repelled by it. Also, all touching should be unambiguous: clearly, touch has sexual connotations for some people.

When we communicate verbally with others, we tend to stand or sit close to them. How near we stand or sit is determined by a number of factors – the level of intimacy we have with them, our relationship with them and whether or not we are dominant or submissive in that relationship (Brown, 1965). In the health-care professions, people tend to be in a dominant position *vis à vis* their patients and clients and tend to stand closer to them than would be the case in ordinary day-to-day relationships.

It is useful to imagine that we are surrounded by an invisible bubble, the threshold of which can only be crossed by certain other people. If people accidentally break through the bubble and touch us, they tend to withdraw quickly to avoid embarrassment to both parties. The issue of proximity to others needs close consideration. We need to become aware of how close or distant we like to be in relation to others. We need also to note other people's preferences and to be sensitive towards them. One useful way of judging this distance between you and the other person is to allow the other person to set that distance. In other words, you invite the other person to draw up a chair or you allow them to determine where they will stand in relation to you and not vice versa. Once again, as we become more self-aware, so we gain more insight into the needs and wants of others.

One of the clearest indicators of our inner experience is facial expression. Frowns and smiles do much to convey the feelings that are being experienced inside. It is important that facial expression and speech are congruent or matched. We have all experienced the person who says that they are cheerful or upset but whose facial expression suggests otherwise. Bandler and Grinder (1975) note that for the purposes of clear communication, three aspects of our outer behaviour must match: general body position, content of speech and facial expression. If two or more of these are mismatched then our communication will be confused and confusing. Thus if we say that we are cheerful but shrug our shoulders and have an unhappy expression, the message will be unclear. We can do a lot to improve our communication on this level. It is insufficient just to say what we mean. We must be *seen* to mean it as well.

Two issues become clear from this brief analysis of the outer aspects of self. We can become aware of our use of speech, eye contact, touch, proximity to others, gesture, facial expression and non-linguistic aspects of speech as a means of deepening our understanding of ourselves. Also, by becoming conscious of how we use those verbal and non-verbal behaviours, we can use them more skilfully to enhance our contact with others. We can increase our interpersonal skills by intentionally using ourselves as instruments. Heron uses the expression 'conscious use of self' (Heron, 1977) to convey this concept. This is not to say that we need to become robotic and artificial but that in caring for others we can more precisely use our 'selves' as instruments of communication.

THE INNER EXPERIENCE

The inner, private experience in this model may be divided into four aspects of mental functioning – thinking, feeling, sensing and intuiting – and the experience of the body. Clearly, the division of these aspects into two groups is artificial as both mental and physical events are interrelated. As Searle (1983) points out, a mental event is also a physical event. To think that it is not is to perpetuate the old philosophical problem of mind/body dualism. This is sometimes known as Cartesian dualism after the philosopher René Descartes, who believed that mental and physical events could be considered separately. Today, the tendency is towards healing this split and interest continues to develop in holistic medicine which treats the mind and body together. As we have already noted, any concept of the self must take into account the mind and the body as a totality.

The thinking dimension

In this model, thinking refers to all the aspects, logical and otherwise, of our mental processes. A moment's reflection on thinking will reveal that it is not a linear process. We do not think in sentences or even in a series of phrases. The process is much more haphazard than that. The technique known as 'free association' used in psychoanalysis demonstrates the apparently random nature of some of our thinking. In free association the individual verbalizes whatever comes into her mind, without any attempt at censoring or stopping the flow. Try to do this. The process is always difficult and sometimes impossible. The reasons for this are outlined in the psychoanalytical literature and such theory can offer insights into the genesis and nature of thought processes. Clearly, not everybody wants or can afford psycho-analysis but its ideas can be useful in attempting to understand thinking.

Arguably, the domain of thinking is more dominant in certain individuals. Certainly, thinking is highly rated in our culture and the education system sometimes seems to concern itself only with this mode. The domains of feeling, sensing and intuiting are usually less well catered for. In the health professions, however, we are concerned with all sorts of feelings, from pain to anxiety, from depression to elation. Understanding these requires the use of dimensions other than thinking. On the other hand, it is obviously important that we all develop the thinking aspect. If we are to progress as a research-based profession and if we are to be able to demonstrate critical awareness, we must be able to think clearly. We must also be able to appreciate when feeling gets in the way of thinking, as well as vice versa.

The feeling dimension

Feeling in this model refers to the emotional aspects of the person: love, sadness, joy, happiness, etc. Heron (1977) argues that there are four dominant aspects of emotion that are frequently denied and repressed in our culture: anger, grief, fear and embarrassment. He argues that anger can be expressed through loud sound and shouting, grief through tears, fear through trembling and embarrassment through laughter. He argues further that such expression of emotion (or catharsis) is a healthy process. Heron claims that we live in a non-cathartic culture and the general tendency is to encourage people to control rather than to express emotion. As a result, we all carry round with us a pool of unexpressed emotion which distorts our thinking and stops us functioning fully. If we can learn to express some of this bottled-up emotion, and methods of doing this will be discussed later, then we can become more open to experience, less fearful and anxious and we can exercise more self-determination and autonomy. Part of becoming self-aware entails discovering and exploring the emotional dimension.

Health-care professionals must deal with other people's emotions and there is a positive link between the way in which we handle our own emotions and the way in which we handle those of others. If we understand and can appropriately express our own anger, fear, grief and embarrassment, we will be better able to handle them in other people. In caring for others, we must get to know ourselves better.

Certainly other people's emotions affect us and stir up our own, unexpressed emotions. Try this simple experiment. Next time a programme on television moves you near to tears, turn off the set and allow yourself to cry. As you do so, reflect on what it is you are crying about. It is highly likely that the issue causing the tears is a personal one, not directly related to the television programme. Most people carry around with them this unexpressed emotion, just beneath the surface. Health-care professionals who work in particularly emotionally charged environments – children's wards, intensive therapy units, psychiatric units and so forth – may want to consider self-help methods for exploring their own hidden emotions. Co-counselling, discussed in the next chapter, is one such method and others are discussed by Bond (1986) and Bond and Kilty (1982). Alternatively, consider going to the cinema as a means of emotional release … what do most people go to the cinema for? To cry, to allow themselves to get frightened or to laugh. The cinema and to a lesser extent, the theatre, concerts and sporting events offer 'natural' release valves for people's pent-up emotion.

The sensing dimension

The sensing dimension in the model refers to inputs through the five special senses – touch, taste, smell, hearing, sight – and also to proprioceptive and kinaesthetic sense. Proprioception refers to our ability to know the position of our bodies and thus to know where we are in space. We do not, for instance, need to think about our body position most of the time. We are fed that information by bundles of nerve fibres know as proprioceptors. Kinaesthetic sense refers to our sense of body movement. Again, this is not something we normally have to think about.

We can make ourselves aware of any of the senses. Another simple experiment will demonstrate this. Stop reading for a moment and pay attention to everything that you can hear. Take in all the sounds around you, the more subtle as well as the more obvious. In doing so, notice how much of this one particular sense is normally passed over and how many sounds are usually filtered out of consciousness. At times it is vital that our senses are selective and that extraneous sounds, images, smells and so on are banished from awareness. On the other hand, often that filtering mechanism becomes too efficient and we filter out or fail to notice many sounds and sights that are around us all the time. We live half asleep.

In developing an awareness of our senses, we can begin to notice the world again. Just as importantly, we can begin to notice each other again. In developing our sense of sight, for instance, we can begin to notice subtle changes in other people's expressions, body postures and other aspects of non-verbal communication. Without that awareness we may miss a considerable amount of essential interpersonal information. In health care, the value of such awareness is clear. Health-care professionals need to be observant. It is not always so clear *how* health-care professionals are supposed to become observant. Like any other skills development, learning to notice takes time and practice. The redeeming feature is that it is a skill which the individual can develop for herself. In a way, it is simply a matter of remembering to notice. Eventually, such awareness or 'staying awake' becomes part of the person.

The intuitive dimension

The intuitive dimension is perhaps the most undervalued. Intuition refers to knowledge and insight that arrive independently of the senses. In other words, we just 'know'. Ornstein (1975), who studied the literature on the differences between the two sides of the brain, identified intuition with the right side. He argued that the two sides have qualitatively different functions. The left side is concerned with cognitive processes and with rationality. The right is more to do with holism, creativity and intuition. If Ornstein is right, the implication is that if the intuitive aspect is developed further (along with creativity) then both sides of the brain will function optimally. Ornstein argues that the present Western culture is dominated by the left-brain approach to education and development. He calls for an educational system that honours creativity and intuition alongside the development of rationality.

Perhaps we neglect intuition through fear of it or concern that it may not be trusted. On the other hand, it is likely that we all have 'hunches' that, when followed, turn out to be 'right'. Many aspects of health care require the health-care professional to be intuitive. Sometimes, in order to empathize with another person, we have to guess at what they are feeling. Sometimes we seem to 'know' what they are feeling. Certainly, group work and counselling depend to a fair degree on this intuitive ability. Carl Rogers, founder of client-centred counselling, noted that when he had a hunch about something that was happening in a counselling session, it invariably helped if he verbalized that intuition (Rogers, 1967). Using intuition consciously and openly takes courage and sometimes it is wrong. On the other hand, used in tandem with more traditional forms of thinking, it can enhance the health-care professional/patient relationship in a way that logic, on its own, never can.

THE EXPERIENCE OF THE BODY

The third aspect of the model of self-awareness is the experience of the body. If the mind and body are directly interrelated, in fact inseparable, then any mental activity will affect the body and vice versa.

It is easy to talk as though the mind and body *were* separate. Indeed, we do not *have* a mind/body, we *are* our mind/body. Everything that we refer to as being part of our mind and body is part of our selves. Expressions such as 'I'm not happy with my body ...' or 'I've got that sort of mind ...' indicate how easy it is for us to dissociate ourselves from either the body or the mind.

Coming to notice body feelings takes time and patience. Of course, appreciation of inner bodily experiences is limited to some degree by the supply of sensory nerve endings to certain aspects of the body. Some parts are better served than others. On the other hand, it is easy to lose touch with those bodily sensations of which we *may* become aware. Before you read any further, just take a moment to notice what is going on inside your body. What do you notice? Are there areas of muscle tension? Are the muscles of your stomach pulled in tightly? Can you become aware of your breathing? Are you breathing deeply into your stomach or is your breathing light and shallow? What happens when you make small changes to your body? What happens when you relax sets of muscles or change your breathing?

All the information that can be gleaned from the body can enable us to appreciate something about our psychological status. Muscle tension, for example, may be the first we know of the fact that we are anxious. Learning to 'listen' to the body in this way can help us to more accurately assess our true feelings about ourselves and others.

Wilhelm Reich (1949), a psychoanalyst who was particularly interested in the mind/body relationship, advanced the notion of 'character armour'. Reich maintained that our emotional feelings could become trapped within muscles and consequently affect posture and movement. He suggested that direct manipulation of those muscles could release the feelings trapped within them with characteristic emotional catharsis. Such manipulation has become known as Reichian bodywork and can be a powerful and effective means of developing self-awareness through direct body contact.

Other methods of this sort which involve direct physical contact include rolfing (Rolf, 1973), bioenergetics (Lowen, 1967) and Feldenkrais (Feldenkrais, 1972), three bodywork methods that have developed out of Reich's original formulation. Less dramatic but equally valid methods of body/mind exploration include massage, yoga, the martial arts, certain types of meditation, the Alexander technique (Alexander, 1969), dance and certain types of sport.

All these methods can enhance awareness of self through attention to changes in the body and thus create insight into psychological states. They can also aid the development of awareness of body image. Observations of people in everyday life will reveal how frequently people walk around with lop-sided shoulders, a stooping gait or even with the two sides of their face showing different expressions. Often, too, they seem to be totally unaware of these things. Bodywork methods can enable the individual to develop greater physical symmetry and balance, better posture, improved breathing and a healthier physical status, generally. All aspects of health care call for psychological and physical stamina and are taxing on the mind/body. These methods in combination with more traditional approaches to self-awareness can lead to a powerful and healthy approach to self-care. Perhaps burnout, so frequently a problem of occupations that depend upon a high degree of human contact, can be prevented effectively through this mix of attention to the body and mind.

SELF-AWARENESS

A model of the self has been outlined which takes account of the inner and outer aspects of the concept and which has attempted to marry the mind and body. The question now arises: what is self-awareness?

A first point that needs to be made is that we are *not* discussing 'self-consciousness', in the everyday sense of the word. To be self-conscious is to be embarrassed by ourselves, to be painfully aware of being observed by others. Sartre (1956) describes this well when he suggests that under the scrutinizing gaze of the other person, we are turned into an object, a 'thing'. It is our response to being treated in this way that causes us to become self-conscious. For the very self-conscious person, this sense of being treated as an object is exaggerated by that person herself. In being too acutely aware of other people's attention, she imagines herself to be more acutely scrutinized than is actually the case. It is rather like having someone watch us undertaking a skill such as giving an injection. We tend to (a) become deskilled by their watching us and (b) imagine that they are being highly critical. Self-consciousness is a bit like this. It tends to make you awkward and tends to make you feel criticized. This is true, for example, of the adolescent who imagines (usually falsely) that they are being looked at with highly critical eyes. Their own sense of insecurity is projected onto the world and they imagine that others view them as harshly and as critically as they view themselves.

Clearly, such self-consciousness is more of a hindrance than a help when it comes to relating to others, as any acutely shy person knows. Yet such self-consciousness is far removed from self-awareness and may indicate a false or exaggerated self-concept.

Self-awareness refers to the gradual and continuous process of noticing and exploring aspects of the self, whether behavioural, psychological or physical, with the intention of developing personal and interpersonal understanding. Such awareness is probably best not developed for its own sake; it is intimately bound up with our relationships with others. To become more aware of and have a deeper understanding of ourselves is to have a sharper and clearer picture of what is happening to others.

In this sense, it is a process of discrimination. The more that we can discriminate ourselves from others, the more we can understand our similarities. If we are unaware and blind to our own selves then we are likely to remain blind to others. A rather crude illustration may help to drive this point home. If I buy a red sweater, I immediately notice how many other people are wearing red sweaters, a fact of which I was not aware before the purchase. In noticing that fact about others I can also notice other things about them. And so, if I let it, the process escalates. I can notice more subtle differences between persons but also their similarities. The point is that the process begins with me. I must first examine myself.

Such a process of examination requires patience and honesty. It is easy to fall into the trap of *interpreting* thoughts, feelings and behaviour, rather than (initially at least) merely noticing them. That interpretation logically comes after we have gathered the data, after we have clearly described to ourselves our present status. This stage of self-awareness training may be likened to the assessment stage of the diagnostic process. Information about the self is gathered in order to develop a clearer picture, before any attempt is made to problem solve, decide upon changes or identify reasons for the way we are.

This approach may be described as *phenomenological* (Spinelli, 1989). Phenomenology is a branch of philosophy that is concerned with attempting to describe things as they appear to be without recourse to making value judgements about them. Thus, in the human context, a phenomenological approach to self-awareness training would concern itself purely with describing aspects of the self as they surface and become known. Such an approach demands that we suspend judgement on ourselves. Instead of telling ourselves that 'this bit of me is OK ... this bit is bad and needs to be changed', we merely note that *it is as it is*. Once we have more data at our disposal, the answer to the question 'why?' may become self-evident. Jumping to hasty conclusions may either wreck the project altogether because we are disenchanted or make us harshly critical of ourselves. Certainly, the road to self-awareness is not an easy one to tread, but the phenomenological approach can make it bearable. After all, if we don't accept ourselves, who will? If we don't accept ourselves, will we accept other people?

This method of description rather than interpretation is of great value in group settings and in counselling. When experiential learning is discussed in the next chapter, the notion of the phenomenological role of the facilitator is described. In this role, the facilitator of the group does not attempt to offer interpretations of what is happening in the group but limits herself to descriptions of events and of behaviours and encourages other group members to do the same. In the context of counselling, the phenomenological approach also pays dividends. If we can stand back and avoid interpreting what it is we think our clients are saying, we give them the chance to make their own interpretations. This attitude towards counselling is known as the client-centred approach (Rogers, 1967; Burnard, 1989). It is argued that the only person who can make a valid interpretation of her behaviour is the person herself.

DEVELOPING SELF-AWARENESS

There are various ways of developing self-awareness. Some involve introspection and some entail involvement with and feedback from other people. Any course leading towards self-awareness must contain both facets: the inner search and the observations of others. Introspection by itself can lead to a one-sided, totally subjective view of the self. It is difficult, if not impossible, for the person working on her own to transcend herself and take the larger view. In order to balance that subjective view, we need the views of others.

Before examining some of the methods of introspection and group work, it is useful to note one simple method of enhancing self-awareness: the process of noticing what we are doing, the process of self-monitoring. All that is involved here is that you stay conscious of what you are doing, as you do it. In other words, you 'stay awake' and develop the skill of keeping your attention focused on your actions, both verbal and non-verbal. Such a process, whilst easy in theory, can in practice be quite difficult. It is easy to become distracted by inner thoughts and preoccupations so that our actions become automatic and unnoticed, even robotic.

All such explorations can be carried out in isolation, with another person or in groups. To explore the self in the company of another person can be a rewarding and economical method, in that the time available can be equally divided between the two people. This is a process by which two people who are trained as co-counsellors meet and spend equal time in the roles of counsellor and client. Co-counselling is a self-awareness method which is taught by various trainers in colleges and extramural departments of universities.

Those learning co-counselling are taught, first, to listen to each other very carefully, not to judge what the other person is saying and not to offer advice. They can, however, make certain interventions that draw the other person's attention to verbal slips, emphases and so on. The following is an example of two people holding a co-counselling session. The extract is from one half of the session in which the first person who talks is in the role of 'client' and the other is in the role of 'counsellor'. After an agreed amount of time, the people will switch roles and the 'client' will become 'counsellor' to the other person. Notice that much of the dialogue is about the counsellor letting the client verbalize and work through his own thoughts and feelings.

'I'm feeling very stressed at the moment. No, not *very* stressed but stressed. I'm not sure what that's all about.'
'You're not sure ...'
'Well, some of it is to do with work. I'm very busy at the moment with some difficult clients. Why are these clients difficult? Are they difficult or do I see them as difficult? One of them, I know, reminds me of myself! That's a painful thought but it's true, I think.'
'You're smiling'.

'Yes. It's ironic, really, I talk to him about all sorts of things that I think he should do but don't do any of them myself. It's a bit hypocritical, really. I'm embarrassed at the thought, I suppose. I need, though, to consider in what sorts of ways he is *different* to me.'

'In what sorts of ways?'

'First, he is older than me. He is married and I am not. He is a different person. It's an odd thing to say but that is important. We are *not* the same person.'

'In what other ways are you different?'

'He is physically different to me. He looks different. He has a temper, though. And when he gets mad, he reminds me of myself.'

'How else is he similar to you?'

'He has the same temperament. No, I don't know him well enough to know whether or not that's true. I think I *like* him. Which is a relief. I thought, for a moment that I saw him as so similar to myself that I wouldn't. That's encouraging and I'm beginning to be able to separate him off from myself. That's important, I think.'

Co-counselling, then, is a method of quiet exploration in the supportive presence of another person. The 'counsellor' does not act in the traditional counselling role but is more supportive, with occasional, client-centred counselling interventions. It can be used to relieve stress, to develop counselling skills and to enhance self-awareness. Co-counselling is fairly easily learned, as a series of skills, and economical to carry out. It does, however, take commitment on the part of the co-counselling practitioners to keep going. It is, like many fairly new ideas, easy to start or initiate but not so easy to continue as a long-term project. However, the rewards for those who do carry on with it are considerable, even if it is only used as a method of peer support amongst health-care colleagues.

Other methods of self-awareness training include the use of role play, social skills training, meditation and assertiveness skills training. These methods are well documented in the literature (see, for example, Kagan, 1985; Bond, 1986; Hargie, Saunders and Dickson, 1987; Burnard, 1989) and courses in these forms of training are frequently organized by women's groups, growth centres and extra-mural departments of colleges and universities.

In health-care professional education and training, the use of video can enhance self-awareness by allowing students to view themselves as if from another person's point of view. Such training, however, should always be voluntary. Some people find the use of video a gross invasion of personal territory and the method should be used with discretion.

As we have noted, work on the body via Reichian bodywork, yoga, tai chi, the martial arts and sport all have their place in self-awareness development not only for their effects on the body but also for their limit-testing capacity. A quieter, more reflective approach is the use of journals or diaries and these can help to monitor self-awareness development alongside educational development.

Probably the ideal is a combination of a variety of approaches: introspection, group work, active and passive. In this way, the self is studied in all its aspects and in a variety of contexts, As we have noted, the 'self' is not a static once-and-for-all thing but an entity that is constantly changing depending, amongst other things, on the people we are with. The eclectic approach is also healthier in that it encourages the combination of sport and exercise alongside meditation and more reflective practices. It also allows for normal social relationships to develop alongside periods of solidarity. No one ever became self-aware by shutting themselves away from the rest of the world. Also, it is important that self-awareness development has a practical end – the enhancement of interpersonal relationships and skills.

SELF-AWARENESS AND THE HEALTH-CARE PROFESSIONAL

Having explored the concept of self and examined some methods of self-awareness development, the question remains: why develop self-awareness anyway?

In the first instance, to discover more about ourselves is to differentiate ourselves from others. If we cannot differentiate between our own thoughts and feelings and those of others, we may blur our ego boundaries, our sense of ourself as an independent, autonomous being. Also, if we constantly blur the distinction between 'you and me' we risk not recognizing the other person's independence and autonomy. When ego boundaries are blurred, we lose the sense of whose problem is whose. With self-awareness we can learn to distinguish between our problems and those of others. This is particularly important in sensitive areas such as psychiatry and care of the dying person. Real involvement and care in these fields also involves (almost paradoxically) the ability to detach ourselves a little in order to get things into perspective. If we cannot engage in this distancing we risk being drawn into other people's problems to such a degree that we can no longer help them. Their problems have become ours.

To become self-aware is also to learn conscious use of the self. We become agents; we are able to choose to act rather than feeling acted upon. We learn to select therapeutic interventions from a range of options so that the patient or client benefits more completely. If we are blind to ourselves we are also blind to our choices. We are blind, then, to caring and therapeutic choices that we could make on behalf of our patients.

Once we can combine two aspects – differentiation from others and an increased awareness of the range of therapeutic choices available to us – we can be more sensitive to the needs and wants of others. We can even choose to *forget ourselves* in order to give ourselves more completely to others. No longer do we run the risk of getting sucked into other people's problems, nor do we confuse our thoughts and feelings with those of our patients. We can offer therapeutic distance with therapeutic choice.

Interpersonal interventions such as counselling and group facilitation require that we exercise some self-awareness. All that has been discussed in the above paragraphs is particularly true when we are trying to help people in these particular sorts of therapeutic situations. In Part Two of this book, both counselling skills and group facilitation skills are explored. It is a vital prerequisite that alongside the development of such skills, self-awareness continues to develop. Skills development without self-awareness tends to encourage a stilted and unnatural presentation of self. Without self-awareness, the person appears merely to have a set of skills 'tacked on' to her; those skills are not used sensitively or awarely but in a robotic and automatic way.

PROBLEMS IN SELF-AWARENESS DEVELOPMENT

It is worth repeating the point made at various stages throughout this chapter that the aim of self-awareness development is to enable us to increase our interpersonal skills. The path to such awareness is, however, fraught with problems. First is the problem of egocentricity. It is possible to become caught up in the idea of understanding the self to the degree that it becomes an end in itself. This tends to lead to the person becoming self-indulgent and self-centred. Clearly such positions are not compatible with altruism or concern for others. Second, it is possible for those who develop self-awareness to believe that they have discovered insights that set them apart or even make them better than other people. A sign of such development is sometimes the loss of a sense of humour. Life becomes very earnest.

True self-awareness, however, tends to lead to a lightness of touch and a sense of humility at the sheer vastness of the task in hand. To continue with that task, it is important that the person maintains (and exercises) a sense of humour in order to keep sight of the 'larger canvas'. Certainly the best run self-awareness groups are those that offer a 'light' atmosphere. If the atmosphere becomes too heavy and earnest, it is likely to put everyone off. It is certainly not conducive to easy and frank self-disclosure.

Linked to this is the problem of the self-awareness group facilitator becoming something of a 'guru' figure. As people find things out about themselves, they sometimes tend to imagine that the group facilitator has special qualities that allow this to happen. As a result, those people tend to set the facilitator up as some sort of heroine. Sometimes the facilitator believes in this image too and ends up acting out the role of guru.

Again, caution and humility are keywords. Both group members and facilitator should remember that the facilitator is human, like everyone else. I use the word 'she' here, but in my experience (and for whatever reason) it is nearly always men who either set themselves up in the guru role or are set up in it by their groups.

Next comes the issue of voluntariness. Self-awareness cannot be forced upon people. Facilitators of self-awareness groups would do well to exercise what Heron (1977) calls the voluntary principle. This is a principle invoked at the beginning of any self-awareness training course and repeated at intervals throughout such a course that no one at any time will have pressure exerted on them to take part and that everyone takes part in any exercise of their own free will. If self-awareness is about developing autonomy and the exercise of choice, it is important that such autonomy and choice begin with deciding whether or not a given exercise suits the person at this time. Accepting and respecting other people's frailties, their reserve and their choice not to disclose aspects of themselves until they are ready are all part of the process of facilitation. Such understanding on the part of the facilitator will do much to increase the confidence of group members and to create an atmosphere conducive to self-understanding.

Finally, there is a much more radical problem with the whole idea of self-awareness. If we consider the two words we will realize that both of them are *abstractions*. Neither self nor awareness has concrete reality. We cannot 'point' to either of them. We cannot directly observe another person's nor our own 'self'. This, in turn, makes it difficult to argue for our being aware of a self, either in ourselves or in others. In this sense, then, the words 'self' and 'awareness' are simply ways of trying to talk about things that cannot readily be apprehended. If this is the case, there is a real danger of *reification*, of treating those abstractions as though they had concrete reality. If we reify, in this case, we start to believe we really do have a 'self' and that we can, by extension, become 'aware' of it.

We can simplify the issue a little if we say something like 'When I talk about self, I mean those elements of my personality that are to do with identity, those things that make me different and similar to other people'. This being the case, it seems reasonable that we should be able to say that we can be aware of some of those things. We should be cautious, though, about being too *definite* about notions of self and self-awareness. The idea that such awareness can help in therapeutic relationships is a popular one but, given that we are dealing with abstractions or 'ways of talking', there is little empirical evidence that such awareness (if it is possible) helps in relationships. The common-sense view might be that 'to know ourselves is to know more about others'. A more measured view might be that this proposition has yet to be verified. Further, some would argue that there are no means by which it could be verified.

Recently, I met a lecturer in a health-care college who had developed a scale for 'measuring' self-awareness in students' essays. It started from zero, which was an indication that the student lacked any sort of self-awareness and ended at 10 which indicated that the student had a considerable degree of awareness and an understanding of the dynamics of personal relationships. Clearly such scales are impossible to validate and cannot be reliable. Any scale of this sort fails on at least three counts:

1. what it 'means' to reach one of the criteria on the scale;
2. how it might be possible to recognize when a student did or did not fulfil one or other of the criteria;
3. there are, presumably, far too many variables from which to judge a person's written work in terms of self-awareness or lack of it.

The whole business of scoring someone on a scale of this sort involves an impossible degree of value judgement. Perhaps, in the end, it might be argued that any debate about the degree to which one is or is not self-aware involves such value judgements. This creates considerable difficulties if we want to reach some sort of agreement, between different people, about the nature and degree of self-awareness. We must continue to remain cautious.

Another problem with the concept of self is that it is often *individualistic*. 'Selves' are often talked of as if they are self-contained and to do only with the individual who 'has' that self. Another argument might be that we are always 'selves-in-relation': we cannot experience ourselves without reference to other people. I am 'me' because I can recognize the fact, more or less, of my difference to you. Some would argue, further, that there is no such thing as an 'individual self' and that we exist only as part of a larger social group or that the idea of an individual self is not a particularly useful one given that we are social beings.

Another view of self is that 'self' is not a continuous experience, that we do not have a fluid and developing sense of self at all. From this point of view, as Kurt Vonnegut (1969) put it, 'You are what you pretend to be. So be careful *what* you pretend to be'. In other words, we are simply 'making ourselves up' as we go along. This is, perhaps, the extreme of the existential position. The past does not necessarily bear any particular relation to the present. We are, at any given time, what we find ourselves to be. This approach (or lack of approach) to self is also reminiscent of an exercise that Bertrand Russell set his students. He used to ask them 'Prove to me that the world and everything in it, including our memories, was not invented yesterday'. Perhaps that which we call 'self' is not as continuous as we would like to believe. On the other hand, it might be difficult, from this point of view, to explain how we know who we are when we wake up each morning. For, certainly, most of us seem to have little difficulty in recognizing ourselves as we come out of a deep sleep, except that it does seem that we have to give the issue some thought: we have to *remember* who we are. Harold Brodkey (1991), at the start of one of his novels, describes a boy waking up:

Anyway, sometimes it seems a shame to leave one's dreams. Maybe it's because real life is hard. I don't, as a rule, have strong opinions about those matters any more than, when I first awake, I don't know quite who I am or where I am; I don't remember what I am *supposed to look like*.

T.S. Eliot wrote that 'we die to each other daily'. Perhaps, to some degree, we also die to ourselves.

PRESENTATION OF SELF

You are an instrument of communication. What you wear, what you say, the way that you say it – all of these communicate who you are to others. We have at least two choices. One is not to take any notice of the how and the what of personal communication. The other is to choose how we communicate. Heron (1977) refers to this as 'conscious use of the self'. In the following questionnaire you are invited to reflect on aspects of self-presentation. During the process, try to make decisions about what and how you need to change (if at all). If you are someone who frequently thinks about their presentation of self, the activity will not be too difficult. If you are someone who infrequently thinks about who and what you are, then the process may be less easy.

Presentation of Self Questionnaire

Work through the following questions and think about the way you present yourself to others.

Clothes

Do you have different sorts of clothes for work and for home?
If so, how do you make decisions about what sorts of clothes to buy for each situation?
Do you consciously strive for a particular style?
What sort of style is it?
When did you last change the style?
Why do you adopt it?

Introductions

How do you introduce yourself to others?
How do you introduce yourself on the telephone?
How do you introduce other people to friends and colleagues?
Is it something you find easy or difficult?
How could you improve your introductions?

Holding a conversation

Are you a good listener?
What do you *do* while you listen?
Are you a 'sentence finisher' when others are talking?
Do you think you talk too much?
Are you shy in conversations?
To what degree do you self-disclose?
How do you handle other people's self-disclosure?
What do you do when you find yourself becoming emotional in a conversation?
What are you like at handling other people's emotion?

Ending conversations

What do you do when you want to finish a conversation?
How do you finish a phone conversation?
Do you find that people keep on talking to you even though you think you have indicated that you have to stop?
What do you need to do to improve the way that you finish a conversation?

Non-verbal communication

Do you look at people when you talk to them?
Are you comfortable making eye contact with other people?
In what situations are you *not* comfortable making eye contact?
What do you do with your hands when you talk?
How do you stand? Are you upright, slightly slouched, uncomfortable …?
What position do you adopt when you are sitting down? Do you cross your legs, fold your arms …?
Do you smile very much?
Do you tend to frown?
How close or distant do you sit or stand in relation to other people?
Have you ever felt uncomfortable in relation to personal space?
Do you ever touch the other person when you speak?
Would you say that you were a 'high toucher' or a 'low toucher'?

Content of conversations

Is conversation a serious business to you?
Do you gossip?
Do you prefer light or heavy conversations?
Is a sense of humour important to you?
Do you talk about yourself a lot?
Do you allow others to talk about themselves?
Which do you prefer, talking or listening?

Your values

What things are most important to you?
Why are they?
In what ways do your values affect your behaviour and the way that you live?
Do you respect people with values different from your own?
How do you handle conflict over values?
Do you ever act against your values?

SUMMARY

We all need to become self-aware in order to offer all we can to our clients, patients and colleagues. This chapter has discussed some ways of developing self-awareness.

References

Alexander, F.M. (1969) *Resurrection of the Body*, University Books, New York.

Bandler, R. and Grinder, J. (1975) *The Structure of Magic, Vol I*, Science and Behavior Books, San Francisco, California.

Bannister, D. and Fransella, F. (1986) *Inquiring Man*, 3rd edn, Croom Helm, London.

Bond, M. (1986) *Stress and Self-Awareness*, Heinemann, London.

Bond, M. and Kilty, J. (1982) *Practical Methods of Coping With Stress*, Human Potential Research Project, University of Surrey, Guildford, Surrey.

Brodkey, H. (1991) *The Runaway Soul*, Vintage, London.

Brown, R. (1965) *Social Psychology*, Collier Macmillan, London.

Buber, M. (1958) *I and Thou*, Scribner, New York.

Burnard, P. (1989) *Teaching Interpersonal Skills: A Handbook of Experiential Learning for Health Professionals*, Chapman & Hall, London.

Feldenkrais, M. (1972) *Awareness Through Movement*, Harper & Row, London.

Hargie, O., Saunders, C. and Dickson, D. (1987) *Social Skills in Interpersonal Communication*, 2nd edn, Croom Helm, London.

Heron, J. (1970) *The Phenomenology of the Gaze*, Human Potential Research Project, University of Surrey, Guildford, Surrey.

Heron, J. (1977) *Behaviour Analysis in Education and Training*, Human Potential Research Project, University of Surrey, Guildford, Surrey.

Jung, C.G. (1938) Psychology and religion, in *Collected Works, Vol 2*, Routledge & Kegan Paul, London.

Jung, C.G. (1978) *Selected Writing*, Fontana, London.

Kagan, C. (ed.) (1985) *Interpersonal Skills in Nursing*, Croom Helm, London.

Kelly, G. (1955) *The Psychology of Personal Constructs* (2 volumes), W. W. Norton, New York.

Laing, R.D. (1959) *The Divided Self*, Penguin, Harmondsworth.

Lowen, A. (1967) *Betrayal of the Body*, Macmillan, New York.

Maslow, A. (1972) *Motivation and Personality*, Harper & Row, London.

Myerscough, P.R. (1989) *Talking With Patients: A Basic Clinical Skill*, Oxford Medical Publications, Oxford.

Ornstein, R.E. (1975) *The Psychology of Consciousness*, Penguin, Harmondsworth.

Reich, W. (1949) *Character Analysis*, Simon and Schuster, New York.

Rogers, C.R. (1967) *On Becoming a Person*, Constable, London.

Rolf, I. (1973) *Structured Integration*, Viking Press, New York.

Rowan, J. (1989) The self: one or many? *The Psychologist: Bulletin of the British Psychological Society*, **7**, 279–81.

Sartre, J.-P. (1956) *Being and Nothingness*, Philosophical Library, New York.

Searle, J. (1983) *Philosophy of Mind*, Cambridge University Press, Cambridge.

Simpson, M. (1996) *It's a Queer World*, Vintage, London.

Spinelli, J. (1989) *The Interpreted World*, Routledge, London.

Vonnegut, K. (1969) *Mother Night*, Gollancz, London.

Skills check: Part One

Sit quietly and reflect on the skills that have been discussed in this section. How many of them are applicable in your health-care setting? To what degree do you feel that you have had training in those that are applicable?

Now ask yourself the following questions.

- To what degree is my writing effective?
- Do I enjoy writing?
- How could I improve it?
- Am I generally assertive?
- In what situations am I *not* assertive?
- To what degree am I self-aware?

PART TWO

Communication and Clients:
Therapeutic skills

Introduction

All health professionals have a therapeutic role. The process of helping or caring for others means that we engage in talking, counselling or advising as part of our everyday work. Part Two examines some of the specific skills that can be called 'therapeutic'.

Chapter 4 explores that most important of all skill, listening and paying attention to another person. This skill, like any other, can be learned and improved upon. The point of this chapter is to reflect on the elements that go towards improving listening and to identify various blocks to listening. We can all learn to listen better.

Counselling has been variously defined. Some see it as part of a managerial function. Others see it almost exclusively as having to do with psychotherapy. Chapter 5 identifies a range of aspects of counselling in health care and considers some of the specific skills of counselling.

Chapter 6 focuses on group work. How do you organize and facilitate groups? What are the stages that most groups go through? The aim of this chapter is to identify the practical and theoretical issues that need to be addressed by anyone planning to set up and run a therapeutic group. The skills involved may also be useful to those running other sorts of groups: support groups, case conferences, management groups and so on.

This section, then, considers a range of *therapeutic* communication skills. They link with the educational ones identified in Part One but also stand on their own.

Listening skills

4

Listening and attending are by far the most important aspects of being a health-care professional. Everyone needs to be listened to. Unfortunately, most of us feel that we are obliged to talk! Unfortunately, too, 'overtalking' by the health-care professional is least productive. If we can train ourselves to give our full attention to and really listen to the other person, we can do much to help them. First, we need to discriminate between the two processes: attending and listening.

ATTENDING

Attending is the act of truly focusing on the other person. It involves consciously making ourselves aware of what the other person is saying and what they are trying to communicate to us. Figure 4.1 demonstrates three hypothetical zones of attention. The zones may help to further clarify this concept of attending and have implications for improving the quality of attention offered to the client.

Zone one represents the attention being fully focused 'outside' ourselves and on the environment around us or, in the context of counselling, on the client. When we have our attention fully focused 'out' in this way, we are fully aware of the other person and not distracted by our own thoughts and feelings.

There are some simple activities, borrowed from meditation practice, that can enhance our ability to offer this sort of attention. Here is a particularly straight-forward one. Stop reading this book for a moment and allow your attention to focus on an object in the room: it may be a clock, a picture or a piece of furniture – anything. Focus your attention on the object and notice every aspect of it – its

THE EXTERNAL WORLD	THE INTERNAL WORLD
	Zone two: Attention focused on inner thoughts and ideas. Perception is based on 'reality' or, at least, on what we perceive as reality.
Zone one: Attention 'out' and focused on the outside world and on the client. The whole of the counsellor's attention is caught up with the client and listening is intense.	
	Zone three: Attention focused on 'fantasy': the counsellor 'invents' ideas, histories, explanations. Perception is based on what is *imagined* to be the case. In this zone, the counsellor develops *theories* about the other person.

Figure 4.1 Three possible zones of attention.

shape, its colour, its size and so forth. Continue to do this for at least one minute. Notice, as you do this, how your attention becomes fully absorbed by the object. You have focused your attention 'out'. Then discontinue your close observation. Notice what is going on in your mind. What are your thoughts and feelings at the moment? When you do this, you shift your attention to zone two: the 'internal' domain of thoughts and feelings. Now shift the focus of your attention out again and onto another object. Study every aspect of it for about a minute. Notice, as you do this, how it is possible to consciously shift the focus of your attention in this way. You can will yourself to focus your attention outside yourself. Practice of this conscious process will improve your ability to fully focus attention outside yourself and onto the client.

If we are to pay close attention to every aspect of the client, it is important to be able to move freely between zones one and two. In practice, what probably happens in a counselling session is that we spend some time in zone one, paying full attention to the client, and then we shuttle back into zone two and notice our reactions, feelings and beliefs about what they are saying, before we shift our attention back out. The important thing is that we learn to gain control over this process. It is not until we train ourselves to consciously focus attention 'out' in this way that we can really notice what the other person is saying and doing.

Zone three in the diagram involves fantasy: ideas and beliefs that bear no direct relation to what is going on at the moment but concern what we think or believe is going on. When we listen to another person, it is quite possible to think and believe all sorts of things about them. We may, for example, think 'I know what he's really trying to tell me. He's trying to say that he doesn't want to go back to work, only he won't admit it ┬ even to himself!'

When we engage in this sort of 'internal dialogue' we are working within the domain of fantasy. We cannot 'know' other things about people, unless we ask them or, as Epting (quoting the personal construct theorist George Kelly) puts it: 'If you want to know what another person is about, ask them, they might just tell you!' (Epting, 1984). We often think that we do know what other people think or feel, without checking with that person first. When we do this, we are focusing on the zone of fantasy: we are engaged in the processes of attribution or interpretation. The problem with these processes is that, if they are wrong, we develop a very distorted picture of the other person! Our assumptions naturally lead us to other assumptions and if we begin to ask questions directly generated by those assumptions, our counselling will lack clarity and our client will end up very confused!

A useful rule, then, is that if we find ourselves within the domain of fantasy and we are 'inventing' things about the person in front of us, we stop and if necessary check those inventions with the client to test the validity of them. If the client confirms them, all well and good: we have intuitively picked up something about the client that he was, perhaps, not consciously or overtly telling us. If, on the other hand, we are wrong, it is probably best to abandon the fantasy altogether. The fantasy, invention or assumption probably tells us more about our own mental make-up than it does about that of our client! In fact, these 'wrong' assumptions can help us gain more self-awareness. In noticing the wrong assumptions we make about others, we can reflect on what those assumptions tell us about ourselves.

Awareness of focus of attention and its shift between the three zones has implications for all aspects of counselling. The health-care professional who is able to keep attention directed out for long periods is likely to be more observant and more accurate than one who is not. The health-care professional who can discriminate between the zone of thinking and the zone of fantasy is less likely to jump to conclusions about their observations or to make value judgements based on interpretation rather than on fact.

What is being suggested here is that we learn to focus directly on the other person (zone one) with occasional moves to the domain of our own thoughts and feelings (zone two) but that we also learn to attempt to avoid the domain of fantasy (zone three). It is almost as though we learn to meet the client as a 'blank slate': we know little about them until they tell us who they are. To work in this way in counselling is, almost paradoxically, very empathic. We learn, rapidly, not to assume things about the other person but to listen to them and to check out any hunches or intuitions we may have about them.

Being able to focus on zone one and have our attention focused out has other advantages. In focusing in this way, we can learn to maintain 'therapeutic distance'. We can learn to distinguish clearly between what are the client's problems and what are our own. It is only when we become mixed up by having our attention partly focused on the client, partly on our own thoughts and feelings and partly on our fantasies and interpretations that we begin to get confused about what the client is telling us and what we are 'saying to ourselves'. We easily confuse our own problems with those of the client.

Second, we can use the concept of the three domains of attention to develop self-awareness. By noticing the times when we have great difficulty in focusing attention 'out', we can learn to identify points of stress and difficulty in our own lives. Typically, we will find it difficult to focus attention out when we are tired, under pressure or emotionally distressed. This can come to serve as a signal that we need to stop and take stock of our own life situation. Further, by allowing ourselves consciously to focus 'in' on zones two and three – the process of introspection – we can examine our thoughts and feelings in order to further understand our own make-up. Indeed, this process of self-exploration seems to be essential if we are to be able to offer another person sustained attention.

If we constantly 'bottle up' problems we will find ourselves distracted by what the client has to say. Typically, when they begin to talk of a problem of theirs that is also a problem for us, we will suddenly find ourselves pondering on our own problems and not those of the client! Regular self-examination can help us to clear away, at least temporarily, some of the more pressing personal problems that we experience.

Such exploration can be carried out in isolation, in pairs or in groups. If done in isolation, meditative techniques can be of value. Often, however, the preference will be to conduct such exploration in pairs or groups. In this way, we gain further insight through hearing other people's thoughts, feelings and observations and we can make useful comparisons between other people's experiences and our own.

There is a variety of formats for running self-awareness groups, including sensitivity groups, encounter groups, group therapy and training groups. Such groups are often organized by colleges and extramural departments of universities but they can also be set up on a 'do-it-yourself' basis. Ernst and Goodison (1981) offer some particularly useful guidelines for setting up, running and maintaining a self-help group for self-exploration. Such a group is useful as a means of developing self-awareness, as a peer support group for talking through counselling problems and also as a means of developing further counselling skills. Trying out new skills in a safe and trusting environment is often a better proposition than trying them out with real clients!

LISTENING

Listening is the process of 'hearing' the other person. This involves noting not only the things that they say but also many other aspects of communication. Given the wide range of ways in which one person tries to communicate with another, this is further evidence of the need to develop the ability to offer close and sustained attention, as outlined above. Three aspects of listening may be noted. Linguistic aspects of speech refer to the actual words that the client uses, the phrases they choose and the metaphors they use to convey how they are feeling. Attention to such metaphors is often useful as metaphorical language can often convey more than conventional use of language (Cox, 1978).

Paralinguistics refer to all those aspects of speech that are not words themselves. Thus, timing, volume, pitch and accent are all paralinguistic aspects of communication. Again, they can offer us indicators of how the other person is feeling beyond the words that they use. Again, however, we must be careful of making assumptions and slipping into zone three, the zone of fantasy. Paralinguistics can only offer us a possible clue to how the other person is feeling. It is important that we check with the client the degree to which that clue matches with the client's own perception of the way they feel.

Non-verbal aspects of communication refer to body language: the way that clients express themselves through the use of the body. Thus facial expression, use of gestures, body position and movement, proximity to the health-care professional, touch in relation to the counsellor, all offer further clues about the client's internal status beyond the words they use and can be 'listened' to by the attentive health-care professional. Again, any assumptions that we make about what such body language 'means' need to be clarified with the client. Ekman and Friesen (1969) identified five different functions of non-verbal behaviour:

1. supporting or complementing the verbal meaning of an utterance, such as pointing to the bathroom down the hall while explaining to a family member where it is located;
2. regulating the flow of the interaction, as in touching someone to get their attention or backing away to end a conversation;
3. signalling specific meanings understood by members of one's culture, usually with head, arm or hand signals. Examples are waving, shrugging or nodding;
4. conveying idiosyncratic habits, which bear little relationship to verbal content, such as holding your chin in your hand when in deep thought or fidgeting with a pencil when you talk to someone;
5. expressing emotion, generally through facial expressions, but also through body posture and distance.

There is a temptation to believe that body language can be 'read', as if we all used it in the same sort of way. Reflection on the subject, however, will reveal that body language is dependent to a large degree on a wide number of variables: the context in which it occurs, the nature of the relationship, the individual's personal style and preference, the personality of the person 'using' the body language and so on. It is safer, therefore, not to assume that we 'know' what another person is 'saying' with their body language but to treat it as a clue and to clarify with the client what they mean by their use of it. Thus it is preferable, in counselling, to merely bring to the client's attention the way they are sitting or their facial expression, rather than to offer an interpretation of it. Two examples may help here. In the first, the health-care professional is offering an interpretation and an assumption.

I notice from the way that you have your arms folded and from your frown that you are uncomfortable with discussing things at home.

Notice that, in this example, the health-care worker is immersed in zone three, the domain of fantasy. She is *imagining* what is going on rather than seeking clarification.

In the second example, the health-care professional merely reflects to the client what she observes and allows the client to clarify their situation.

I notice that you have your arms folded and that you're frowning. What are you feeling at the moment?

Grove (1991) also suggests other ways in which we can increase our awareness of the meaning of another person's non-verbal communication.

1. We can become more attuned to non-verbal leakage, those non-verbal cues that the communicator is apparently unaware of that contain information about their feelings or attitudes. For example, a patient who is nervously wringing their hands communicates to us their anxiety, even though their words may deny it. Being aware of subtle non-verbal behaviours helps us 'read between the lines' in interpreting another's emotional state.
2. We can become aware of clues to deception, instances in which verbal and non-verbal behaviours do not match. Rather than relying solely on a person's words for meaning, we need to note any discrepant non-verbal cues that contradict what they say. Markers of deceitful communication include decreased eye contact, increases in foot, hand and leg movements, increases in idiosyncratic non-verbal gestures that are not correlated in the verbal message.
3. We need to focus on the total context of the interaction in order to more accurately perceive non-verbal behaviours. We cannot correctly attribute meaning to a single isolated non-verbal cue; for example, a frown might mean disapproval, concern, confusion, anger or despair, depending on the situation and the complex set of communication cues emitted from a communicator. Important contextual features include the communication setting, what is being said and why, the history of the communicator's relationship and how a communicator customarily behaves.

LEVELS OF LISTENING

The skilled health-care professional learns to listen to all three aspects of communication and tries to resist the temptation to interpret what she hears. Three levels of listening may be identified.

1. *Linguistic aspects.* Words, phrases, metaphors, etc.
2. *Paralinguistic aspects.* Timing, volume, pitch, accent, 'ums and ers', fluency, etc.
3. *Non-Verbal aspects.* Facial expression, use of gesture, touch, body position, proximity to the health-care professional, body movement, eye contact, etc.

The first level of listening refers to the idea of the health-care professional merely noting what is being said. In this mode, neither client nor health-care professional are psychologically very 'close' and arguably the relationship will not develop very much.

In the second level of listening, the health-care professional learns to develop 'free-floating' attention. That is to say that she listens 'overall' to what is being said, as opposed to trying to catch every word. Free-floating attention also refers to 'going with' the client, of not trying to keep the client to a particular theme but of following their conversation wherever it goes. She also 'listens' to the client's non-verbal and paralinguistic behaviour as indicators of what the client is thinking and feeling. Faced with this deeper level of listening, the client feels a greater amount of empathy being offered by the health-care professional. The health-care professional begins to enter the frame of reference of the client and to explore their perpetual world. She begins to see the world as the client experiences it.

In the third level of listening, the health-care professional maintains free-floating attention, notices non-verbal and paralinguistic aspects of communication but also notices her own internal thoughts, feelings and body sensations. As Rollo May (1989) notes, it is frequently the case that what the health-care professional is feeling, once the counselling relationship has deepened, is a direct mirror image of what the client is feeling. Thus the health-care professional sensitively notices changes in herself and gently checks these with the client. It is as though the health-care professional is listening both to the client and to herself and carefully using herself as a sounding board for how the relationship is developing. Watkins (1978) has described this process as 'resonance' and points out that it is different to that of empathizing.

> Rogers says that empathy means understanding of the feelings of another. He holds that the therapist does not necessarily himself experience the feelings. If he did, according to Rogers, that would be identification, and this is not the same as empathy. Resonance is a type of identification which is temporary.

The use of resonance needs to be judged carefully. Whilst it does not involve interpreting or offering a theory about what the client is feeling, it does offer a particularly close form of listening which can make the client feel listened to and fully understood. It is notable, too, that in these circumstances, the client will often feel more comfortable with periods of silence as they struggle to verbalize their thoughts and feelings. Arguably, they allow these silences because they sense that the health-care professional is 'with them' more completely than at other levels of listening. The net result of this deeper level of listening is that a truly empathic relationship develops. The client feels listened to, the health-care professional feels she is understanding the client and a level of mutuality is achieved in which both people are communicating, both rationally and intuitively.

USE OF 'MINIMAL PROMPTS'

Whilst the health-care professional is listening to the client, it is important that she shows that she is listening. An obvious aid to this is the use of what may be described as 'minimal prompts' – head nods, yes, mm and so on. All of these indicate that 'I am with you'. On the other hand, overuse of them can be irritating to the client, particularly the thoughtless and repetitive nodding of the head – the 'dog in the back of the car' phenomenon! It is important that the health-care professional, at least initially, is consciously aware of her use of minimal prompts and tries to vary her repertoire. It is important to note, also, that very often such prompts are not necessary at all. Often, all the client needs is to be listened to and they appreciate that the health-care professional is listening, without the need for further reinforcement of the fact.

It should also be noted that there are cultural differences in the ways that minimal prompts are used. North Americans, for example, tend to use the acknowledgement 'uh-huh' as another person talks. People in the UK do not so readily use this form of intervention. While there is no harm in trying out something new, it is important not to sound too stilted by 'borrowing' another culture's minimal prompts.

BEHAVIOURAL ASPECTS OF LISTENING

Another factor in the process of listening is the behaviour the health-care professional adopts when listening to the client. Egan (1990) offers the acronym SOLER as a means of identifying and remembering the sorts of counsellor behaviour that encourage effective listening.

* sit Squarely in relation to the client.
* maintain an Open position.
* Lean slightly towards the client.
* maintain reasonable Eye contact with the client.
* Relax!

First, the health-care professional is encouraged to sit squarely in relation to the client. This can be understood both literally and metaphorically. In North America and the UK it is generally acknowledged that one person listens to another more effectively if she sits opposite or nearly opposite the other person, rather than next to them. Sitting opposite allows the health-care professional to see all aspects of communication, both paralinguistic and non-verbal, that might be missed if she sat next to the client.

Second, the health-care professional should consider adopting an open position in relation to the client. Again, this can be understood both literally and metaphorically. A 'closed' attitude is as much a block to effective counselling as is a closed body position. Crossed arms and legs, however, can convey a defensive feeling to the client and counselling is often more effective if the health-care professional sits without crossing either. Having said that, many people feel more comfortable sitting with their legs crossed, so perhaps some licence should be used here! However, sitting in a 'knotted' position with both arms and legs crossed should be avoided.

It is helpful if the health-care professional appreciates that leaning towards the client can encourage them and make them feel more understood. If this does not seem immediately clear, next time you talk to someone, try leaning away from the other person and note the result!

Eye contact with the client should be reasonably sustained and a good rule of thumb is that the amount of eye contact that the health-care professional uses should roughly match the amount the client uses. It is important, however, that the health-care professional's eyes should be 'available' for the client, that she is always prepared to maintain eye contact. On the other hand, it is important that the client does not feel stared at nor intimidated by the health-care professional's glare. Conscious use of eye contact can ensure that the client feels listened to and understood but not uncomfortable.

The amount of eye contact the health-care professional can make will depend on a number of factors, including the topic under discussion, the degree of 'comfortableness' she feels with the client, the degree to which she feels attracted to the client, the amount, nature and quality of the client's eye contact and so forth. If the health-care professional continually finds the maintenance of eye contact difficult, it is perhaps useful to consider talking the issue over with a trusted colleague or with a peer support group, for eye contact is a vital channel of communication in most interpersonal encounters (Heron, 1970).

Finally, it is important that the health-care professional feels relaxed while listening. This usually means that she should refrain from 'rehearsing responses' in her head. It means that she gives herself up completely to the task of listening and trusts that she will make an appropriate response when she has to. This underlines the need to consider listening as the most important aspect of counselling. Everything else is secondary to it.

Many people feel that they have to have a ready response when engaged in a conversation with another person. In counselling, however, the main focus of the conversation is the client. The health-care professional's verbal responses, although important, must be secondary to what the client has to say. Thus all the health-care professional has to do is sit back and listen intently. Easily said but not so easily done! The temptation to 'overtalk' is often great but can lessen with more experience and with the making of a conscious decision not to make too many verbal interventions.

All of these behavioural considerations can help the listening process. In order to be effective, however, they need to be used consciously. The health-care professional needs to pay attention to using them and choose to use them. As we have noted, at first this conscious use of self will feel uncomfortable and unnatural. Practice makes it easier and with that practice comes the development of the health-care professional's own style of working and behaving in the counselling relationship. No such style can develop if the health-care professional does not first consciously consider the way she sits and the way she listens.

In summary, it is possible to identify some of those things which act as blocks to effective listening and some aids to effective listening. No doubt the reader can add to both of these lists and such additions are useful in that they are a reflection of your own strengths and limitations as a listener.

Blocks to Effective Listening

- The health-care professional's own problems
- The health-care professional's stress and anxiety
- Awkward/uncomfortable seating
- Lack of attention to listening behaviour
- Value judgements and interpretations on the part of the health-care professional
- Attention focused 'in' rather than 'out'
- 'Rehearsals' inside the health-care professional's head

Aids to Effective Listening

- Attention focused 'out'
- Suspension of judgement by the health-care professional
- Attention to the behavioural aspects of listening
- Comfortable seating
- Avoidance of interpretation
- Judicious use of minimal prompts

Blocks to talking

Just as we may put up barriers that indicate to patients or clients that we are not really listening to them, there are also various things that may make it difficult for patients and clients to talk. Referring to doctor/patient relationships, Myerscough (1989) suggested that reticence to talk may be due to the following.

- The presence of a third party – a nurse, a student or even an accompanying relative. They should, if necessary, be asked to leave the room.
- Sometimes the fact that the doctor is also the family doctor may inhibit an adolescent from speaking freely.

- The patient may fear that revealing their complaints will lead to the realization of their worst fears: a diagnosis of serious disease, admission to hospital, an operation.
- A reluctance to take up the doctor's time with concerns that the patient may feel are undeserving of his time and attention: 'You are always a very busy man, doctor, and there are several folk still waiting to see you'.
- Embarrassment or shame about the nature of the complaint. This might apply to a wide range of disorders, but especially to those with a sexual association: venereal disease; other genital complaints; drinking problems; pregnancy in the unmarried, widowed or separated; impotence.
- Cultural barriers. For example, many Asian women find it difficult to discuss personal or marital problems with a male doctor or even with a strange female doctor. A youthful or venerable-looking doctor may be seen as an unsuitable confidant if he obviously belongs to a different generation from the patient.

We might note, in passing, some of the assumptions that Myerscough makes in his list: that in the fourth point, the doctor is necessarily a man and that the patient refers to other patients as 'folk' and that in the final point, Myerscough is able to refer to a 'venerable-looking' doctor. In the final point, too, Myerscough seems to find it odd that an Asian woman might not be able to talk to a doctor – *even* a 'strange female doctor'. These points may seem minor but they also betray certain values and beliefs about health-care professional/patient relationships. When we consider listening to others, we should also think about listening to ourselves.

ACTIVE LISTENING

This term is sometimes used to imply the fact that listening is not simply a passive act of sitting there and hearing what the other person says. As we have seen, active listening involves a range of behaviours ranging from non-verbal ones to prompts. Active listening may also include short sentences or phrases which encourage the other person to say more. The following is an example of someone engaging in active listening. Note how the 'conversation' is totally focused on the talker.

'I get worried sometimes. I feel I'm not going to be able to cope and that I will cave in. What worries me most is that my wife won't be able to cope either. I mean, if I cave in, why should she cope?'
'Both of you not coping ...'
'Well, in some ways, she is stronger than I am. I accept that. Well, I sort of accept that. Sometimes I think that I should be stronger than I am and that I should be able to sort of take more responsibility for myself. And for her. She seems to shoulder everything, really.'
'What does she have to shoulder?'
'Me, the kids, the money problems. Everything, really. I suppose, if I'm

honest, I have had quite a cushy time of it up to now. I'm like a big child, myself, in a way. And that makes it worse. I wish I didn't realize that, really. It would be easier.'

'It would be easier if you didn't see yourself as a big child ...'

'Sometimes it would. Sometimes. ... I suppose the other point is that, if I can *realize* it, I could do something about it. I suppose I have to accept that I *am* an adult and not a child. I have to take some responsibility. Perhaps I should stop whining a bit and just get on with life. I should be able to do that. I mean, having realized that I am a bit weak, I should be able to do something about it'.

'You feel that you can?'

'I think so. I need to focus more on Jane than on myself. On Jane and the children. Yes. I think I have become a bit too self-centred. I read, some- where, that it pays to be 'outward looking' and not to be too introspective. I think I will try that. It can't hurt to try.'

Although this almost shades into counselling, it is also an example of active listening. The health professional in this example is not offering advice, making suggestions or directing the conversation in any particular way. All that she is doing is 'staying with' the client and concentrating hard on listening to what he is saying. Her short, verbal interventions make this evident to the client, who carries on talking and works things out for himself. In some ways, then, active listening involves an act of faith.

WHAT DO PEOPLE *MEAN* WHEN THEY TALK?

All listening involves a degree of *interpretation*. We can view levels of interpretation in various ways. At one level, for example, we might check that we are clear about the meanings of words that the speaker is using. At another, we may add a layer of *theoretical* interpretation to what is said. Thus if we were followers of Freud, we might view what is said from a series of Freudian interpretations. However hard we try to be 'neutral' in listening, the quest remains an impossible one. Trying to establish *absolute* meanings for what is said is nigh on impossible. To take this a little further – and perhaps a lot further – we might do well to consider the approach taken in *postmodernism*. The discussion that follows can also be applied to other sections of this book, from the chapter on counselling to the one on computing. For in all cases of communication, we are forced to ask 'What does this *mean*?'.

The question of meaning has been addressed by postmodernists. Postmod- ernism is, in some ways, a popular theoretical mood in sociological and aesthetic circles (Lyon, 1994). The term 'mood' is used advisedly: postmodernism, by nature, is difficult to pin down and even more difficult to define. It is best viewed, obliquely, by allusion and by reference to other markers.

What is postmodernism? First, we can say what it is *not*. It is not a 'school' or a series of propositions. In this respect, it is not dissimilar to another philosophical tradition that is difficult to pin down: existentialism (Sartre, 1956, 1973). Because both are against 'systems building' and the development of the 'grand theory', both suffer the problem of definition and, to some degree, lack of popularity. Their vagueness and abstraction are sometimes a reason for their dismissal. Further, their concentration on subjective experience and multiplicity of meaning makes their tenets difficult to support or dismiss with any authority or clarity.

The idea of the postmodern suggests a 'modern' period and an ending of that period. Lyon (1994) suggests that the modern period began with the Enlightenment and ended some time in the 1950s or 1960s. The modern period was characterized by many writers as involving, above all things, a sense of forward propulsion, a notion of *progress*. This, it might be argued, reached its peak in the 1960s, particularly in the field of architecture. 1960s architecture, generally condemned in the present day, is characterized by the Brave New World feeling of the times. Progress, even a 'revolution', was almost taken for granted. This theme of 'development' and 'progress' can be traced throughout the centuries back to the Age of Enlightenment.

Perhaps the most important feature of postmodernism is the idea that *progress is not inevitable*. Postmodernists, if they would define themselves as such, might argue that we look in all directions, not merely forward, when we view the world, its theories and its content. In the past, so the argument goes, we looked towards the future as though it was inevitably going to be better than the present. This, again, was exemplified in the 1960s American and USSR space programme. That programme not only involved the search for new horizons (including horizons on the moon) but also the anticipation of a whole range of benefits to humanity.

The 'dream' of progress, was, however, not fulfilled. The Brave New World never arrived and postmodern thinkers were forced to the conclusion that advances were not necessarily and inevitably forward looking. Thinking, culture, art and almost everything else did not progress in a linear fashion. There might be regression as well as progression and the lack of linear development made the idea of progress in theory a difficult one. This provoked the second idea: the possibility of multiple meanings.

Postmodernists argue that 'all is surface'. An example that is readily available to the author might serve here. Before sitting down to write this section, I drove along a section of a motorway in which roadworks were taking place. After the roadworks was a sign that read: 'The Welsh Office apologizes for any incon-venience caused'. Reflection on this sign will reveal that there is no 'Welsh Office apologizing' nor any single person who is being apologetic. Further reflection suggests that the sign is almost meaningless: *no one* is 'sorry' for the inconvenience. The sign is merely a social nicety. Alternatively, we might want to say, the sign is *full* of meaning. It encapsulates the (perhaps abstract) notion of a local government 'concerned' with its image and with the views that drivers might have of it. So we might argue that the sign is both 'surface' *and* open to interpretation. What we will never achieve, however, is any sense of the 'true' meaning of the sign. Arguably, we cannot even go back to the person who devised the idea of the sign and ask for an explanation: theirs will merely be *another* view and not *the* view. Again, to the driver who speaks no English or Welsh, the sign will mean nothing, except perhaps that it will register as 'a sign'. In this sense, all we have is 'marks on paper': the characters themselves have no hidden meaning.

We may choose to 'interpret' and impute 'deeper' meanings into human behaviour and events but, in the end, we are forced to confront that it is we who bring the meanings to behaviours and events and therefore there are no *absolute* meanings to those behaviours and events. All we can acknowledge is that anything can be viewed from a multiplicity of positions. The most obvious and clear examples of this can be seen in the interpretation of art and music. There are, clearly, no final arbiters of what is and what is not 'good art' or 'good music'. Each of us is left to decide, for ourselves, what we do or do not 'like' and what 'interpretation' we make of a painting or a piece of music.

We can extend this idea to the field of literature. It might be argued that the 'true meaning' of a piece of written text is that which the writer of it intended. However, the issue is far from clear. We might want to try to establish 'what Shakespeare really meant' but the project is doomed. We never have access to Shakespeare and, again, there is no final arbiter of what Shakespeare did or did not mean. Stated more strongly, though, the issue becomes one of the possibility of *multiple meanings*. Each person's reading of Shakespeare (or any other writer) can be different and no one, finally, can say that that reading is 'wrong'. Thus the idea of multiple meanings and the point that the postmodernist writer Lyotard (1983) makes that it is the 'reader who writes the text' become apparent. The reader, the viewer, the listener, makes what they will of a piece of written text, a picture or something that they have heard. According to postmodernism, no writer or artist can complain 'But that's not what I meant!'. For the postmodernist, all meanings are valid. In this sense, then, all types of meaning are 'allowed'. This is, arguably, equally true of conversation. What we 'hear' and what a person 'says' are both open to interpretation or a series of interpretations. It is always going to be difficult to arbitrate over the question of who is right.

To summarize: postmodernism questions the inevitability of progress and acknowledges the possibility of multiple meanings of text. And *text* can be broadly defined as any set of symbols. Thus, music can be text, architecture can be text and the written word can make up text. This, then, is a much broader definition of *text* than has sometimes previously been given. Some examples of 'postmodern' text might be examined here.

Lyon (1994) argues that *Blade Runner* is an example of the postmodern film in that it offers fragmentation, alienation and multiple meanings. In the field of architecture, the postmodern influence can be seen in almost all new shopping precincts. Most of these draw on a wide range of 'influences', from the Ancient Greek to the Victorian to the present-day American. There is, paradoxically, nothing modern about these buildings and yet all draw on a range of references to create something which is immediately recognizable as late 20th century, at least for the moment. However, it seems likely that, in the future, such architecture will be viewed quite differently. It will be 'interpreted' and theories will be developed about what late 20th century architects were 'really' trying to do. And then we are back to the Shakespeare Problem. No one will be able to offer the final or even remotely definitive theory of why such buildings were built. Interpretation, then, becomes an *arbitrary* process. If interpretation is arbitrary, then no ultimate or transcendental theory of interpretation can be claimed. The arbitrariness rules out the possibility of ultimate or 'correct' interpretations.

Another view of 'meaning' is offered by Luoto (1996). He suggests that when someone gives us a verbal message, we internally go through a process of interpretation which can usefully be modelled in steps, as follows.

1. Generate a possible interpretation (representation) for the message. This will be a much fuller representation than just the mere words and will include material from our own experience, our 'map' of the world.
2. Evaluate the representation. The first criterion of evaluation is 'Does this make any sort of sense?'. Further criteria include 'How well does this match my view of the world?' and possibly others.
3. If the evaluation is 'doesn't make any sense' or 'isn't on my map', go back to step 1 to generate another possible interpretation.
4. After generating at least one and possibly several interpretations (representations), take the one that most closely matches our criterion as the 'meaning' of the message.

This, then, is something of the paradox of listening: we must try to listen impartially and fairly objectively but, at the same time, we are always forced to interpret and make sense of what we hear. Listening can never be a 'clean' activity: we can never get to the nub of what people *really* mean, just as, as readers, we can never get to the 'real' meaning of a book. We have to learn to live with this sort of ambiguity and attempt to cope with it. The best we can aim at, perhaps, is a *shared* understanding: in listening to our patients and clients we can try to reach something of a consensus of opinion about what those patients and clients are trying to express.

SUMMARY

The skills of attending and listening are essential ones that can be used in every health professional's job. The skills are clearly not limited only to use within a counselling relationship but can be applied in other interpersonal exchanges. An advantage of developing these particular skills is that becoming an effective listener not only makes for better practice but interpersonal effectiveness and self-awareness are also enhanced.

REFERENCES

Cox, M. (1978) *Structuring the Therapeutic Process*, Pergamon, London.

Egan, G. (1990) *The Skilled Helper*, 4th edn, Brooks/Cole, Pacific Grove, California.

Ekman, P. and Friesen, W.V. (1969) Nonverbal leakage and cues to deception. *Psychiatry*, **32**, 88–106.

Epting, F. (1984) *Personal Construct Counselling and Psychotherapy*, Wiley, Chichester.

Ernst, S. and Goodison, C. (1981) *In Your Own Hands: A Book of Self-Help Therapy*, Women's Press, London.

➤ Grove, T.G. (1991) *Dyadic Interaction: Choice and Change in Conversations and Relationships*, Brown, Dubuque, Iowa.

Heron, J. (1970) *The Phenomenology of the Gaze*, Human Potential Research Centre, University of Surrey, Guildford, Surrey.

Luoto, K. (1996) Sensitivity and e-mail. Psych-couns discussion list. Psych-couns@mailbase.ac.uk. 14.7.96.

Lyon, D. (1994) *Postmodernity*, Open University Press, Buckingham.

Lyotard, J.-F. (1983) Answering the Question: What is postmodernism? in *Innovation/ Renovation*, (eds I. Hassan and S. Hassan), University of Wisconsin Press, Madison, Wisconsin.

May, R. (1989) Answer to Ken Wilber and John Rowan. *Journal of Humanistic Psychology*, **29**(2), 244–8.

Myerscough, P.R. (1989) *Talking With Patients: A Basic Clinical Skill*, Oxford Medical Publications, Oxford.

Sartre, J.-P. (1956) *Being and Nothingness*, Philosophical Library, New York.

Sartre, J.-P. (1973) *Humanism and Existentialism*, Methuen, London.

Watkins, J. (1978) *The Therapeutic Self*, Human Sciences Press, New York.

Counselling skills | 5

AIMS OF THE CHAPTER

The following issues and skills are discussed.

- What is counselling?
- Counselling skills
- Coping with emotional release

DEFINING COUNSELLING

Counselling is the process of sitting and talking to a client, patient or colleague with the intention of helping them to arrive at decisions about how to act. The action element of counselling comes after the counselling session. In a sense, the counsellor rarely sees the outcome of their work. The counselling session may be the place where things get talked about but the action takes place away from that session, in the person's everyday life. In the considerable literature on the topic, counselling has been defined in various ways.

Noonan (1983) took a historical view in order to define counselling and noted its relationship to psychotherapy. He also commented on its relationship to *friendship* and this is an interesting and contentious point.

> Counselling has its beginnings, both historically as an emerging discipline and daily as a popular activity, in many different professions. It fills the gap between psychotherapy and friendship and it has become a recognized extension of the work of almost everyone whose business touches upon the personal, social, occupational, medical, educational and spiritual aspects of people.

It might be argued that those who have appropriate and well-developed friendships might get all they need from those, rather than from counselling. On the other hand, it seems likely that many people lack nurturing friendships and that some form of counselling might fill this gap. Developing this comparison between friendship and counselling, Aptekar's older definition notes the 'private' quality of counselling.

> Counselling can be carried out privately and without the need to call on agency resources ... all that is required is a person who has a problem and one who is willing to share that problem and bring to bear upon it whatever skills he may have, so that a solution may be reached.
>
> (Aptekar, 1955)

Breese (1983) noted the *time factor* involved in counselling and commented on the nature of counselling as a relationship in which people can talk openly and freely – again, perhaps, reflecting the similarities between counselling and friendship.

> [Counselling is] offering a chance to talk freely and openly, individually or in a group in a non-authoritarian atmosphere, on a regular (normally weekly) basis, within a structure of time and place where people have the opportunity a) to be heard and understood; b) to see things from the point of view of others; and c) to gain greater understanding of themselves and others.

In a book exclusively about counselling (Burnard, 1989), I have focused a definition on the need for counselling to involve not only talking but also the need for action. It remains my belief that counselling is essentially a practical activity.

> The process of counselling is the means by which one person helps another to clarify his or her life situation and to decide further lines of action.

The British Association for Counselling, a body which registers counsellors and approves courses of training, describes counselling from a fairly definitely humanistic point of view but has evolved its definition of counselling from:

> The term 'counselling' includes work with individuals and with relationships which may be developmental, crisis-support, psycho-therapeutic, guiding or problem-solving ... The task of counselling is to give the 'client' an opportunity to explore, discover and clarify ways of living more satisfyingly and resourcefully.
>
> (BAC, 1984)

to:

> ... the skilled and principled use of a relationship to facilitate self-knowledge, emotional acceptance and growth, and the optimal development of personal resources. The overall aim is to provide the opportunity to work towards living more satisfyingly and resourcefully. Counselling ... may be concerned with development issues, addressing and resolving personal insights and knowledge, working through feelings of inner conflict or improving relationships with others.
>
> (BAC, 1989)

Burks and Stefflre (1979) defined counselling in terms of its being a 'professional' relationship involving 'trained' people, as follows.

Counselling denotes a professional relationship between a trained counsellor and client. This relationship is usually person-to-person, although it may sometimes involve more than two people. It is designed to help clients to understand and clarify their views of their life-space, and to learn to reach their self-determined goals through meaningful, well-informed choices and through resolutions of problems of an emotional or interpersonal nature.

(Burks and Stefflre, 1979)

This definition highlights the likelihood of counselling taking place between two people although it is less clear what might be meant by a person's 'life-space'.

Richard Nelson-Jones, a writer with wide experience of both doing and teaching counselling, takes the most inclusive view of counselling.

The term 'counselling' is used in a number of ways. For instance, counselling may be viewed: as a special kind of *helping relationship*; as a *repertoire of interventions*; as a *psychological process*; or in terms of its *goals*, or the *people who counsel*, or its *relationship to psychotherapy* .

(Nelson-Jones, 1995)

The client-centred approach to counselling is perhaps the one most widely used today in the caring and health professions and is the one discussed here. However, other, equally effective methods exist, notably the cognitive approach and the more directive and prescriptive approaches described elsewhere (Burnard, 1989).

SOME PROBLEMS WITH COUNSELLING

It is hard to escape references to counselling. After most disasters, news reporters note that 'survivors were offered counselling'. There are numerous telephone helplines which offer help and advice on a whole range of issues. However, in the health professions, there are many issues which disrupt effective communication between patients or clients and health professionals and which can affect the value of counselling. Kreps and Query (1990) identify the following problems in health-care communication, all of which have a bearing on the counselling relationship.

1. *Patient compliance.* Low levels of compliance have been linked to ineffective health-care provider–patient relationships; also, non-compliance has been correlated with poor medical outcomes.
2. *Miscommunication and misinformation.* Ineffective message strategies and failure to seek and utilize feedback contribute to patients' failure to receive the health-care information they need.
3. *Insensitivity* in provider–patient interactions has been linked to low levels of respect, attempts at relational control and inaccurate interpretation of non-verbal messages.

4. *Unrealistic expectations and stereotyping* on the part of both patients and providers have led to misinterpretations of each other's needs and inflexibility in role performance. Patients expect medical personnel to be all-knowing; health-care providers think patients should be unquestionably compliant. These expectations inevitably lead to disappointment, anger and resentment.
5. *Lack of interprofessional understanding and co-operation* is a major problem in health-care delivery. When health-care team members display arrogance and ethnocentrism in their attitudes towards other team members and constantly engage in turf wars, the health-care delivery system suffers.
6. *Ethical and moral questions* concerning informed consent, equal treatment and access to health care, confidentiality, and distorting or withholding information are dilemmas affecting health care delivery. Moral issues involving euthanasia and cultural and religious strictures concerning patient care further complicate the picture.
7. *Dissatisfaction* on the part of both health-care personnel and health-care consumers is linked to other health communication problems, including failure to express empathy, relational dominance and dehumanization.

There are, however, various other questions that remain unanswered. The most important of these is: 'Does counselling work?'. Or, put another way, 'Does counselling make people feel better?'. The aim of this section is to raise a whole range of questions about counselling in health care to enable the formulation of research questions. For if counselling is in need of anything, it is in need of research.

WHAT IS IT?

First, what is counselling? As we have noted above, it is not difficult to put together a range of stipulative definitions. But this in turn raises two other questions. Does counselling differ in any important ways from other sorts of conversation? Does counselling differ from psychotherapy? These are important in establishing *who* counsels and *what sort of training* they have.

If counselling does not differ substantially from other sorts of 'friendly conversation', then the need to find out whether or not it 'works' is less urgent. We do not need research to find out whether or not talking about problems helps people. The fact is self-evident. We all find ourselves talking to spouses, partners, friends and colleagues when we have problems and few of us would need any more 'proof' that it works. We know it works because we have all found it to be the case. Presumably, if talking to other people did not make a difference, we would all have given up the enterprise. Also, from this point of view, counselling clients are self-selecting. Arguably, those who go for counselling are those who find talking about problems beneficial. Those who do not find it beneficial presumably do not seek counselling.

On the other hand, if counselling is nothing more than friendly conversation, we would have to ask questions such as 'Do we *all* do counselling?'. If the answer to that is 'yes', then it would seem that there is little need for counselling training. I suspect that most counsellors would argue that what they do amounts to more than ordinary conversation.

The important question here is what is it that counsellors do that the rest of us, in all other aspects of our lives, do not do? Simply answering that 'we listen' seems inadequate here. Presumably, there are plenty of 'good listeners' amongst the general population who would not call themselves counsellors.

That, then, is the first question and range of subquestions. The second question, raised at the beginning of this section, is 'Does counselling differ from psychotherapy?'. Are counsellors doing very different things to psychotherapists, slightly different things or very similar things? If the latter is the case, do we need a separate name for the activity known as counselling or could all counsellors call themselves psychotherapists? If what counsellors do is very different to what psychotherapists do, what are those differences? Presumably, the fact that two groups of practitioners have sprung up – psychotherapists and counsellors – means that at least some people do see important differences between the two activities.

COUNSELLING AND PSYCHOTHERAPY

McLeod (1994) acknowledges the problem of the counselling/psychotherapy divide and in an important book called *Doing Research in Counselling*, chooses to 'collapse' counselling and psychotherapy together and treat them as similar sorts of things. In doing this, of course, counselling is laid open to the same sorts of criticisms that have been levelled at psychotherapy.

Perhaps the best known criticism of psychotherapy is that made by Masson (1988). After piling up evidence of the 'horrors' perpetrated by some psycho-therapists and after accusing Carl Rogers (father of client-centred therapy) of being the 'bland teaching the unbland how to be bland', Masson comes to the conclusion that all forms of therapy are flawed. He argues that any sort of therapy involves imposing one set of values on another. If you go for therapy, according to Masson, you simply get the therapist's values imposed on yours. This, he argues, is as true of client-centred, non-directive sorts of therapy as it is of the more confrontational sorts.

A much more scathing attack on therapy is made by King-Spooner (1995). In noting the lack of empirical evidence to support the efficacy (or otherwise) of psy-chotherapy, he compares psychotherapy to an animal that is about to become extinct.

Psychotherapy waddles, bloated with self-congratulation, through a benign undergrowth of conferences, workshops, consulting rooms, congenial journals, its strongest characteristics if not its defining expression one of inane amiability.

This 'amiability' may be psychotherapy's and counselling's Achilles heel. For in always adopting a positive and life-enhancing approach to the world, therapists can, arguably, be less than critical. If, as many therapists do, you adopt the view that what matters is another person's point of view and that the best disposition you can hold towards others is an empathic and sensitive one, you can be discouraged from questioning yourself and other people. For to question may be to disagree and therapists, in the main, are not trained to disagree or to be critical. Perhaps therapists need to become more robust, at least with themselves and their discipline. Learning to 'do' therapy within a particular theoretical framework often rules out the possibility of disagreeing with that framework: you either accept it or you do something else. Disagreements, where they occur, most often occur between therapy factions and not within them.

In much earlier attempts at defining psychotherapy as a 'professional' practice, English and English (1958) suggested that psychotherapy was:

> ... the use of any psychological technique in the treatment of mental disorder or maladjustment. The term is very general. It includes 'faith cures', suggestion, hypnosis, psychoanalysis, provision of rest, assurance, advice, consultation designed to relieve anxiety, psychodrama, etc. Nearly always personal consultation is a part of the technique, sometimes the whole of it. The term carries no implications about the seriousness of a disorder ... the duration or intensity of treatment, or the theoretical orientation of the therapist. But the term should be reserved for treatment by a professionally trained person – i.e. by a clinical psychologist, psychiatrist or psychiatric social worker.

What is interesting in this definition, perhaps, is that English and English allude to 'faith cures' but do not include the possibility that all the types of therapy that they identify might also be forms of 'faith cures'. What appears, time after time, in studies of both counselling and psychotherapy is that the important thing is not so much the techniques used by the practitioner but the relationship that develops between the practitioner and the client. We might argue that what the client really looks for is faith in the practitioner. Not blind faith, as in 'this person will cure me', but faith in the idea that 'this person will listen to me and is prepared to help me'.

AN INTERNET STUDY OF COUNSELLING AND PSYCHOTHERAPY

The author conducted a small-scale study using newsgroups on the Internet. The aim of this study was to explore perceived differences between counselling and psychotherapy. A message was posted by the writer on two newsgroups, 'psychiatric-nursing' and 'counselling', inviting group members to submit definitions of counselling and psychotherapy. They were also told of the writer's intention to analyse the responses. It was also noted that a 'summary' of the findings would be posted to the newsgroups at a later date. This was carried out after a reasonable amount of time had elapsed to allow 'late' responses.

There were 26 usable responses to the question. One 'written' response was received through the conventional mail system. One respondent indicated that no part of their response could be used in the analysis without prior permission and this response was excluded from the analysis. The sample could be described as a convenience or opportunistic sample. The nature of the sampling technique means that, as is the case with all qualitative studies, generalizations from the study are not possible or intended.

There were responses from the UK, USA, Canada, Australia, New Zealand and Japan. The text from the e-mail messages was cut and pasted into Word for Windows and then 'cleaned' to remove all headings and unwanted symbols and to standardize the format of the data. E-mail messages arrive in a variety of formats and layouts and these need to be smoothed out before an analysis is attempted. The cleaned text was then transferred to the program *NUD*IST* (Non-numerical Unstructured Data Indexing, Searching and Theory-building). *NUD*IST* is a text management program which helps in the organization and categorization of textual, qualitative data. In the simple analysis offered here, only two categories were used to organize the text: 'definitions of counselling' and 'definitions of psychotherapy'. Finally, the data from *NUD*IST* were transferred back to Word for Windows for the preparation of this report. At a later date, a more detailed and varied analysis will be carried out, again using *NUD*IST* to manage the data.

A number of respondents felt that either there was little difference between counselling and psychotherapy or there was little value in making such a distinction. Some also noted that the discussion had been running for some considerable time. A few felt that the debate was a sterile one. Some respondents also quoted definitions from various bibliographical sources. These have been omitted from this summary.

Counselling

The immediate, here and now, forward-looking focus was identified as a key feature by one respondent.

> I see counselling as being concerned with the 'here and now' and future orientation, whereas psychotherapy is trying to explain behaviours in terms of past remembered and unremembered events.

The 'problem-solving' element of counselling was highlighted by various respondents.

> Counselling is a process to encourage a client to deal with a problem through the help of a counsellor. For this to occur the client is required to talk about their situation. A counsellor will only be able to assist the client to understand the problem if there is effective communication between them. Active listening skills help the counsellor to establish a feeling of respect, empathy and genuineness in the client so that the subconscious protocol is present and counselling can occur.

Counselling, I think, has a similar goal as psychotherapy, which is to assist the client to function 'better' (whatever that means). But counselling to me is a more problem oriented, solution oriented, time limited and fairly acute process. It can be more directive than psychotherapy in that the counsellor has a sense of answers/solutions to problem 1, 2, and 3 (or however many are on the list ...), and moves the client towards those answers/solutions, using a variety of fairly specific techniques (e.g. relaxation training).

I refer to counselling when the presentation is of a person's problem and the response is focused on enabling the person/client to explore or decide solutions to problems. This may include personal insights into the need for more global change and recognition of the potential value of deeper therapy.

The following definition seems to stress the need for closeness and empathy between the counsellor and the client, and the context of the relationship.

At the heart of the counselling process is the communication of ideas from the client to the counsellor. Just as it is necessary to place the problems of the client into the context of their circumstances, it is important to put the words into their context before starting to discuss any quotation.

Quite a different tack was taken by another respondent who offered a 'broader' definition of counselling.

A perception within my sphere of education is that counselling is to be used as a means to enable the student to conform to the norms of the society in which they find themselves. Even the justice system will see counselling in this role in the way it will order offenders to take counselling for their problems. Also there is a tendency to enrol volunteers with minimal experience and training to take on front end counselling ... Counselling would include all the above as well as other interventions. Counselling would then be the practice, and psychotherapy is but one intervention by the counsellor.

Another respondent compared and contrasted counselling and psychotherapy in terms of 'depth' but also acknowledged that the distinction was far from straightforward.

Generally, the convention is that counselling is 'surface' and psychotherapy is 'deep' – as a previous post indicated. This doesn't quite match up with reality (whatever that is). There is also the interesting distinction between counselling, psychotherapy and therapy (minus the psycho-). Behaviour therapy can be quite superficial OR it can effect quite dramatic (and profound) changes (not necessarily intended).Then again people like Windy Dryden [a British writer on counselling and psychotherapy] talk about behavioural and cognitive-behavioural counselling, as well as therapy.

'Distance' and 'closeness' were issues for two respondents and the first of the following suggested that friendship and counselling are virtually synonymous (except, perhaps, in terms of motive). This is disputed by the next respondent.

There is no essential difference between conversation with a friend and counselling, except that the professional counsellor does it better, without bias, and for remuneration.

The essential about counselling is that the counsellor distances him or herself from the subject, to attempt to provide objective evaluation and reflection of the subject's situation. That's why it can be such a difficult situation to 'advise' a friend.

The final quote identifies the perceived 'merging' of counselling with psychotherapy by one respondent and introduces the notion of 'unconscious' thoughts and feelings. It should be noted, too, that many respondents saw considerable similarities between counselling and psychotherapy both in terms of practice and also in terms of the literature. The point was made by one respondent that Carl Rogers described himself both as a counsellor *and* a psychotherapist. This is perhaps most obvious in his collection of essays *On Becoming a Person*.

I believe counselling merges into psychotherapy, but in the latter one makes it overt to the subject that unconscious thoughts and feelings are being explored. As has been intimated in this discussion, the definition lies in the hands of the counsellor/psychotherapist. But I think the therapist has to make a decision on what level the client/therapist interaction is being made overt.

Psychotherapy

The problem-solving side of psychotherapy was again identified under the heading of psychotherapy.

The public perception is that psychotherapy is much more enabling of the person to achieve goals regardless of any understanding of their position and whether the goals are the ones that require to be achieved.

One respondent attempted to identify something of the 'range' of approaches to psychotherapy, thus:

It appears that psychotherapy is a relatively specific intervention and can be limited to concepts and techniques that grew from psychoanalytic models, the client-centred model, and more recently, the communication models. Many intervention approaches can be, and are therapeutic, but would not be psychotherapy in this limited sense. These would include, but not be limited to, educational techniques, persuasion modelling, direct reinforcement of behaviours and guidance.

On the other hand, another respondent suggested that it was 'counselling' that was the 'broader' activity and noted some of the problems with this fact.

> Psychotherapy is often seen as specialist and proactive whilst counselling is a much broader church ... In many ways this breadth has led to a devaluation of the skills of a counsellor as well as a misunderstanding of the role of the counselling process.

One respondent was keen to stress the 'work' and painful elements of psychotherapy.

> Psychotherapy takes time and hard work. It takes commitment on the part of the client to be willing to look at often very painful issues, and I believe it takes great sensitivity and humility on the part of the therapist who can help to guide the client 'safely' through the process.

For one respondent, the difference between counselling and psychotherapy appeared to be the 'length' of the relationship. Psychotherapy was something to be undertaken 'delicately'.

> I think psychotherapy is more introspective for both the client and the therapist, and is an unfolding of a story in a very careful, delicate way. Counselling is a shorter story (still being careful and delicate, of course!) with a more action-driven outcome than psychotherapy. I refer to psychotherapy when the presentation is of the person him or herself with a view to more global exploration of his or her life. The focus then is on aspects of self with a view to personal change or personal insight. This may of course include reflection of the impact of such change on specific problems.

Others saw psychotherapy as being intimately related to self-concept.

> Psychotherapy is – I guess – more concerned with effecting changes which result in a shift in self-concept, identity (or indeed anything connected with the 'self'). Therapy might ... be just about helping people change. Counselling might 'just' be about helping people *feel* differently, although not necessarily behaving differently.

> I see psychotherapy as a specific approach to dealing with issues; an approach that focuses on exploring the inner self of the individual (within the context of individual or group sessions), taking into account the past, the present and the future. The past includes memories, perceptions and dreams of experience. Psychotherapy assists the client in putting all of these pieces into some understandable or at least tolerable framework so that the client can move forward in life. (This sounds a bit pompous, but I can't think of a more simple way to say it ...)

One US respondent made an interesting distinction in that some people in the US are qualified and registered to work as counsellors while they may not be so qualified and registered to work as psychotherapists.

There were various responses to the project itself. Some felt that the discussion was one that had been overemphasized in recent years. Others felt that it was important to continue to try to tease out distinctions between the two. Yet others highlighted the fact that there was considerable overlap between the two activities. This lack of a clear distinction between the two seems to be emphasized by the responses reported above. There were also questions raised about the researcher's motives for carrying out such a project – a not uncommon response to people asking for information.

CLIENT-CENTRED COUNSELLING

Separating counselling out from psychotherapy is difficult. It is probably safe to say that the most frequently described approach to counselling in the literature is *client-centred counselling*. And yet, when we examine the literature related to client-centred counselling we find that all of Carl Rogers' work is described as *therapy* and Rogers consistently described himself as a 'therapist'. It is only in much more recent years that the phrase 'client-centred counselling' has come to be used.

These, then, are the first two questions: 'Is counselling an activity in its own right or is it something indistinguishable from the sorts of conversations we have with friends?'. When we see a counsellor, are we 'buying a friend'? Is counselling the same as psychotherapy or something quite different? If different, what constitutes the difference?

THE MIDDLE VIEW

We may, of course, settle for a 'middle' view on these issues. We may say that 'counselling is rather like a friendly conversation and is related to psychotherapy just as psychotherapy has many of the characteristics of ordinary conversations'. This may be a wonderful piece of fence-sitting or it may be an attempt to settle some differences of opinion.

Once we have clarified what counselling is, we have to return to the question: 'Does it work and if so, why?'. We may want to say that if people have been doing something called counselling for x number of years and if people are employed as counsellors, then that is evidence enough. However, given the current political and economic climate, this is hardly likely to be enough for those who carry out health-care audits. When deciding how to allocate budgets to various services, most health-care managers want hard evidence of the efficacy of health-care interventions. It is unlikely to be enough simply for counsellors to claim 'I *know* it works'. If money is short (and mostly it is) then services for which there is no concrete evidence of their value are likely to be cut. Counsellors, then, like all other health-care workers, need to be clear about their value and be able to demonstrate it.

RESEARCHING COUNSELLING

How might we find out whether or not counselling makes a difference? This is probably the thorniest question of all. The outcome studies that are available are few and far between (McLeod, 1994).

Perhaps the biggest problem lies in filtering out counselling as a discrete variable. After all, counselling, if it works, is likely to be only one of the things that has helped a person. We live surrounded by other people and our lives are constantly changing, as is our health status. To identify counselling as the one thing that 'made a difference' is always going to be difficult.

As another approach to answering the question about efficacy, we might ask clients what they think of the counselling that they receive. This, too, is fraught with problems and often for the same sorts of reasons. If you ask someone 'Is the counselling you are receiving making a difference to you?', the first answer seems likely to be 'yes' (if it was 'no', why would they be continuing with it?). Then, even if they elaborate on that initial answer, how can they tell that it is counselling that is making a difference and not 101 other aspects of their life experience?

Third, we might ask clients, their families and their counsellors to report on the process of counselling. Although we would appear to be piling up evidence through this approach, we are open to the same sorts of criticism. We will never know what it was that made a difference. Was it the counselling or the fact that the families began to talk to each other more? Would they have talked to each other without the counselling? And so on.

And here is the conundrum: we do counselling, we need to know whether or not it works and yet we do not have the means to find out. This leads to the final question: What should we do? Should we acknowledge that our 'intuition' tells us that counselling works? Or, much more radical, should we stop doing counselling until some methods of researching it become available? The latter solution may be radical but it is also the least likely to appeal. We might argue, for instance, that over the centuries there have been many treatments and therapies of proven efficacy which have later been validated by research. The fact that we do not, as yet, have an explanation for how, why or whether counselling works may not be a reason for stopping doing it.

We may, of course, justify using counselling on the grounds that 'people ask for it and say that it helps'. In the end, though, this is unlikely to convince budget holders and is not a particularly good basis for establishing a research platform. In the end, this sort of argument could be used to justify almost anything that was popular.

To return to the beginning of the section: there *are* ways of clarifying some of the issues. If we can be clear about what counselling is and how (if at all) it differs from conversation and from psychotherapy, we may be better placed to find research methodologies. If we are clearer about what we are offering and what it is that we do, then we may be able to formulate working research questions. We need, in other words, to define our terms. We should be prepared, though, to be totally open-minded about the issue. Once we begin to research counselling, we may find that some of it, at least, does not work.

COST EFFECTIVENESS

Although opinions vary as to how the cost effectiveness or otherwise of counselling might be assessed or even if it *should* be assessed, it seems increasingly likely that health-care administration bodies will want to know whether it is more economical to employ a counsellor or another sort of practitioner. In the end, counselling will have to stand its ground alongside all other possible health-care interventions. On the other hand, this will not affect the degree to which all health-care professionals might use counselling skills in their everyday practice. It is one thing to be employed as a full- or part-time counsellor and quite another to use a range of counselling skills as part of another job.

COUNSELLING SKILLS

Counselling skills may be divided into two subgroups: listening and attending and counselling interventions. Listening and attending were considered in the last chapter. This chapter identifies important counselling interventions, the things that the health-care professional says in the counselling relationship.

The term 'client centred', first used by Carl Rogers (1952), refers to the notion that the client is best able to decide how to find the solutions to their problems in living. 'Client centred' in this sense may be contrasted with the idea of 'counsellor centred' or 'professional centred', both of which may suggest that someone other than the client is the 'expert'. Whilst this may be true when applied to certain concrete 'factual' problems, housing, surgery, legal problems and so forth, it is difficult to see how it can apply to personal life issues. In such cases, it is the client who identifies the problem and the client who, given time and space, can find their way through the problem to the solution.

Murgatroyd (1985) summarizes the client-centred position as follows.

- A person in need has come to you for help.
- In order to be helped they need to know that you have understood how they think and feel.
- They also need to know that, whatever your own feelings about who or what they are or about what they have or have not done, you accept them as they are.
- You accept their right to decide their own lives for themselves.
- In the light of this knowledge about your acceptance and understanding of them they will begin to open themselves to the possibility of change and development.
- But if they feel that their association with you is conditional upon their changing, they may feel pressurized and reject your help.

The first issue identified by Murgatroyd is the fact of the client coming for help and needing to be understood and accepted. What we need to consider now are ways of helping the person to express themselves, to open themselves and thus to begin to change. It is worth noting, too, the almost paradoxical nature of Murgatroyd's last point: that if the client feels that their association with you is conditional upon their changing, they may reject your help. Thus we enter into the counselling relationship without even being desirous of the other person changing!

In a sense, this is an impossible state of affairs. If we did not hope for change, we presumably would not enter into the task of counselling in the first place! On another level, however, the point is a very important one. People change at their own rate and in their own time. The process cannot be rushed and we cannot will another person to change. Nor can we expect them to change to become more the sort of person that we would like them to be. We must meet them on their own terms and observe change as they wish and will it to be (or not, as the case may be). This sort of counselling, then, is very altruistic. It demands of us that we make no demands of others.

Client-centred counselling is a process rather than a particular set of skills. It evolves through the relationship that the health-care professional has with the client and vice versa. In a sense, it is a period of growth for both parties, for each learns from the other. It also involves the exercise of restraint. The health-care professional must restrain herself from offering advice and from the temptation to 'put the client's life right for them'.

The outcome of such counselling cannot be predicted nor can concrete goals be set (unless they are devised by the client, at their request). In essence, client-centred counselling involves an act of faith, a belief in the other person's ability to find solutions through the process of therapeutic conversation and through the act of being engaged in a close relationship with another human being.

ROGERS, CLIENT-CENTRED COUNSELLING AND THE ISSUE OF MEANING

Carl Rogers trained in 'classic' psychological style (Kirschenbaum, 1979). At first, he practised what he called 'educational therapy'. His aim was to help families who had 'problem children' to change their situation by his offering the latest 'psychological insights'. His theory, at that time, was that people who were offered clear and up-to-date information would change their behaviour. Then he realized that this did not work. People were, more often, driven by their *own* beliefs about what was and what was not important in their lives. Thus he developed a quite different and, at the time, revolutionary theory. This, in essence, involved encouraging people to talk about their problems and to draw their own conclusions about what the 'meaning' of those problems was. In this way, Rogers suggested that what was important was the *individual's theory about their life*. There were no 'experts' in the human condition. We largely construct our own theories and beliefs about 'how the world is' and act accordingly. This theme has since been taken up by a number of psychological theorists with notable examples being George Kelly (1955) and Guy Claxton (1984). For Rogers, what counted was not what the expert thought but what the client made of their situation.

In this sense, then, Rogers was allowing for multiple constructions of reality. He met clients as 'blank slates'. He did not 'read into' their utterances nor construct theories about why this person was this way at this time. He relied almost entirely on the client developing and exploring their own interpretation of their own situation (Rogers, 1952, 1967).

Rogers later expanded this approach into a general theory of education although this was never as well articulated as his work in the field of therapy (Rogers, 1983). It was Rogers' contention that education should actively involve students in choosing almost all aspects of the educational process. To this end, students might not only choose what to study but how and why that topic might be a useful and interesting one to study. Students' *perceptions* of the world and of the 'knowledge contained in it' were more important than any objectified notion of knowledge. In the end, knowledge itself became a process of negotiation and debate. This in turn could be compared and contrasted with a more classical approach to education, which involved the notion of there being relatively secure 'boundaries' to knowledge and the notion that students should be 'initiated' into such fields of knowledge (Peters, 1969). For Rogers, what was important was that each student's view of the world be accepted as relevant and appropriate. The Rogerian approach to education could be described as *liberal* and was an approach that led to the andragogy of Malcolm Knowles (1975, 1978) and to experiential learning (Burnard 1992, 1995). Experiential learning was later to be incorporated, at least in part, into health-care education, as was the student-centred approach to learning (Allcock, 1992).

In these senses, then, Rogers could be labelled as 'postmodern'. It may be helpful to put a gloss on this claim. First, postmodernism rails against the inevitability of progress. Rogers only partly satisfies this. He accepts that what is important is the acceptance of each person's particular and subjective view of their situation. However, Rogers adds his own, positive ingredient to this idea. He introduces an almost 'moral' suggestion that, in his experience, people left to their own devices could be trusted to make the 'right' decisions. Rogers' world, then, was an almost ideal one: if we could learn to trust each other, we would, through some inbuilt human mechanism, begin to make the appropriate decisions for ourselves and, by implication, for each other. In this sense, Rogers was not particularly postmodern. It is almost as if he cleaned up postmodernism. Whilst the postmodernist would claim that *any* interpretations and decisions were possible – good, bad and indifferent – Rogers might claim that people generally were led in the direction of the 'good' by following an instinctual drive to be right. It might be said, then, that Rogers lost his nerve and abandoned the idea of individuals following their own projects leading to *any* possibility. In this sense, too, there was a large dose of the American in Rogers' work: optimism, positive thinking and the striving to improve.

On the other hand, where Rogers does qualify as a postmodernist is in the fact that he 'allows' for an almost inexhaustible range of possible meanings in the human situation. Unlike Freud, Rogers does not attempt to interpret human behaviour nor bring to it any preconceived notions of how humans might 'work'. Unlike the behaviourists, Rogers does not see humans as programmable and open to manipulation by external forces or loci of control. Instead, he takes a transcendental approach: he suggests that what matters is the individual, human and subjective response to any given situation. He seems to claim to be able to 'stand outside' the experience and situation of others in order not to judge or moralize. This, in turn, leaves Rogers in a curious ethical position. In apparently accepting everything about another human being, he was, presumably, accepting of the 'bad' as well as of the 'good'. For him to maintain his complete acceptance of different world views, he would have to allow that the murderer's point of view is as 'valid' as that of the person who expresses strong religious opinions. He reaches, very quickly, a position of either moral relativism or moral anarchy.

In one sense, Rogers is guilty of a flabby relativism: everything is dependent on the individual's point of view and there are no fixed markers in human behaviour which can lead us to a definitive interpretation of that person's life. The problem with relativism (a state in which everything is dependent on context and situation and in which everything is 'relative' to something else) is that the *relativist position can never be stated*. If we say that 'everything is relative', this is an *absolute* statement! If, on the other hand, we say that 'some things are relative' we are bound to ask 'which ones?'. And then certain things are seen as being not relative. This is the conundrum and paradox of relativism. Ultimately, it may also be the undoing of postmodernism. For the moment, though, it can be argued that Carl Rogers, client-centred counsellor and humanistic educator, was postmodern in a time that is often defined as still being within the modern period (Lyotard, 1983). It might be recalled that Rogers' ideas of the client-centred approach were being formulated in the late 1930s and early 1940s – a period usually defined as being well within the modern period.

A CRITIQUE OF THE CLIENT-CENTRED APPROACH TO COUNSELLING

Philosophically, client-centred counselling has its roots in the existential movement (Sartre, 1956). Rogers adopted this general philosophical position after losing the religious beliefs he held during the early part of his career (Kirschenbaum, 1979). Existentialism involves the notion that people are born as 'blank slates' and only become who they are at a later date. Central to existentialism is the notion of 'existence predating essence'. In Sartre's words:

Man first of all exists, encounters himself and surges up in the world and defines himself afterwards. If man as the existentialists see him is not definable, it is because to begin with he is nothing. He will not be anything until later and then he will become what he makes of himself.

(Sartre, 1973)

Thus, for the existentialist, the only person who can make life decisions for a person is that person themselves. I cannot 'choose' for you, I cannot make up your mind and only you have the power to decide how you will or will not turn out. This is the notion of free will carried to the ultimate extreme, although it should be noted that existentialism only addresses a person's *psychological* freedom. Clearly, a person cannot will to change their height or the social context into which they were born. For the existentialist, the person is the one who shapes their own psychological destiny. What is odd, perhaps, is that this mid-European philosophy of the post-war era was so readily incorporated into an all-American psychotherapy and counselling style.

However, it is evident that existentialism went through a transition in order to become client-centred counselling: it took on board some very American features. The ingredient that Rogers added to this freedom of will was *optimism*. The existentialists tended not to view humans as 'essentially' good, bad or indifferent. Rogers' formulation of the person, however, was closer to that of Rousseau. Rogers claimed that, given the chance, people would always make 'good' decisions (Rogers, 1967). He argued that people were, at base, positive, life asserting and intuitively able to make the right decisions for themselves. All that was required was that the client-centred counsellor kept out of the way of this evolving, positive person and facilitated their growth. Rogers saw people as able to 'grow', although this type of growth was never very clearly defined. Rogers uses the analogy of a bean shoot growing towards the light as an analogy for the person working towards the right set of decisions for themselves. What must always be remembered, however, is that this was only a metaphor. It would be too easy to assume that people really are like the metaphorical bean shoot. Also, it is important to see Rogers' work in the context in which it arose: an economically strong, post-war, optimistic USA in which individualism and liberalism flourished.

The 'optimism' rule of client-centred counselling clearly violates the general rule of free will. If people really are free, then they are free to become anything – good or bad. To argue that people are only 'free to be good' is odd indeed: it is difficult to qualify the concept of freedom. If people are somehow 'programmed' to become good, then they are no longer free agents. Rogers thus 'softened' existentialism and added a large dose of 'pull-yourself-up-by-your-bootstraps' traditional American flavouring.

In order to carry through client-centred counselling to its completion, this belief in the inherent goodness of people is essential. Rogers' only 'commandment' was not to offer advice but to listen and encourage the individual to find their own answers to problems thrown up in counselling. This is only morally acceptable if we truly believe that people are 'good' beneath their current unhappy or distressed state. If, for example, a client discusses violent feelings towards others, we can only *not* intervene if we hold this optimistic view. If we do not hold such a positive view of others, we would, presumably, fear that the other person might act on such feelings and thus feel compelled to advise them not to do so. But Rogers holds the 'no advice' rule right to the end. For Rogers only the individual can find their own way and only the ideas that the client identifies are useful. Any suggestions on the part of the counsellor are seen as an impediment in the healing and growth processes.

However, there seem to be some problems here. First, we might argue that to hold such a positive view of others, in the light of all the confounding evidence of wars, violence, abuse and so on, is naive in the extreme. The evidence that people are 'essentially good' is thin. This is an issue on which various other psychologists and philosophers (including Martin Buber and Rollo May) attacked Rogers. May, for example, accused Rogers of avoiding the 'problem of evil' (May, 1989). Rogers tended to respond to this argument by suggesting that, in his experience, the evidence always pointed to the positive side of human beings. In arguing in this way, Rogers was relying only on his own experience. It might be argued that more evidence was necessary before a general principle of human behaviour was promulgated. In the end, we are left with Rogers' word that people are essentially good and little in the way of evidence.

Once the possibility that people might not be good is raised, the idea that people should *only* be encouraged to follow their own beliefs, feelings and ideas becomes suspect. As we have seen, if we do not hold this underlying optimistic view of people, then advising people to accept very negative or aggressive feelings seems inadequate at best and irresponsible at worst. If, for example, we were counselling a person who discussed a planned murder or suicide, we would have to hold the 'optimistic' belief in people very strongly indeed if we were not to explore possibilities other than murder or suicide.

The second argument against the client-centred approach is one of economy. Rogers wants us to believe that we are all individuals and, as such, are the only ones who can make up our own minds and find our own solutions. However, if this were strictly true, we would have difficulty in empathizing with and understanding each other. Clearly we share many feelings, experiences, thoughts and ideas. I experience love, anger, aimlessness, futility, pleasure and so on and I am able to pass on to you my perceptions of these experiences. If this is the case, then it seems likely that some of the strategies that I use to solve problems may be of use to you. It seems reasonable, therefore, when I find you in trouble, to discuss with you some of the things that have 'worked' for me. At best, you may find something of value in what I say. At worst, you can ignore what I have to say. In a very literal sense, I cannot make your mind up for you. I can, however, give you something to think about and, in the end, you are always at liberty to ignore what I say.

There is a sense in which client-centred counselling offers a great opportunity to reinvent the wheel. All problems are 'individual' and none has been experienced, previously, by another person. Thus, advice and suggestions are not appropriate because no one has ever experienced problems in quite this way before. In a very literal sense, this is true but it is not a particularly important truth. While no one has experienced the world *exactly* as I have experienced it, no doubt many have come very close.

This also, in my view, ignores the common humanity that we share. In many ways, we are more alike than we are different. As I have suggested above, many of the routine (and less routine) experiences that we have are also ones that other people have. Indeed, most of us come to rely on the advice and suggestions of others, not so that we can blindly take that advice or adopt those suggestions but so that we have some fuel for our own problem solving. In everyday life, most of us ask others for their views on what they would do if they found themselves in our position. And, by and large, we listen to what the other person has to say.

The client-centred approach, then, offers an optimistic view of the person which is not backed up by evidence that people really are 'good'. Indeed, it would be possible to look out at the world and come to quite a different conclusion about the 'essence' of people. Also, in eschewing all advice giving, it removes one range of counselling possibilities. It stops us from sharing with the client some of the things that have happened to us. In doing this, it forces the client into the unenviable position of being totally alone in their decision making. It is also disingenuous. The client-centred counsellor has to adopt a 'naive' position in relation to the client. It is as if the client-centred counsellor is saying 'I can't help you here: I have no suggestions as to what you might do: you alone must decide. I will sit with you until you come up with suggestions but it would be wrong of me to prompt you in any way'. This seems to me to be not only dishonest but also uncaring. Part of the business of being human is the ability to share ourselves and our experiences with others. The client-centred approach, however, removes one half of that equation. In the end, we experience ourselves through other people. We depend on other people to tell us who we are. If they offer us no feedback save our own thoughts and feelings reflected back to us, we remain trapped within our own view of ourselves. This can be claustrophobic at best and solipsistic at worst. Nichols (1991) describes what he calls *advisory counselling* which seems to summarize a position in which the counsellor *can* give advice and information:

> The key characteristic [of advisory counselling] is that the main traffic of communication flows from the counsellor, although the communication is modified according to the needs of the person with whom he or she is working. The work includes giving information and advice, shaping attitudes and clarifying present and future medical intentions. The basic context of advisory counselling is, therefore, to do with what the counsellor needs to say. Such work must be conducted in a counselling style though with close attention to the reactions of the person or people involved. It is of critical importance that these reactions are expressed and explored, and thus advisory counselling is essentially interactive.

None of what has gone before is intended to suggest that counselling should involve *only* advice giving. Clearly, advice given in an oppressive and dictatorial way would be of little value. However, it would not be particularly dangerous as it seems unlikely that the client would take advice given in this manner. We can overestimate the effect that we have on others. As in most things, there needs to be a sense of balance. At times it is useful to help people to find their own solutions, without interference. At others, it seems likely that the odd comment or suggestion might trigger new ways of thinking about problems.

The health professional who is able to combine the best of client-centred counselling approaches with a certain sharing of their own experiences seems to strike the balance between helping the client to develop autonomy and leaving the client entirely to their own devices. At its most extreme, the client-centred position turns out to be its own form of tyranny (Masson, 1988). For if I consistently refuse to agree with you, disagree with you or offer any opinion on what you say, then I have you in a very powerful psychological armlock. I appear to be helping you but instead, in standing back from you completely, I force you to confront yourself. This, in turn, can turn out to be its own form of oppression. A more balanced form of counselling might include some elements of the client-centred approach along with some advice, suggestion and information giving.

Given the nature of the health professions, which involve education, information giving and caring, it seems reasonable to argue that such a balanced position should be considered in training health professionals to be counsellors. Also, health professionals, by the nature of their training and experience, do have advice and information that they can usefully share with others. To withhold information and advice in order to satisfy a particular theory of how counselling should be practised may even be negligent. To empower others, we must first rid ourselves of our own dogmas. And client-centred counselling might just have become another – albeit benign – dogma.

It should be acknowledged that the client-centred approach to counselling is not the only one. Other writers on counselling have argued for a more robust and comprehensive approach, including Heron's formulation of a counselling category analysis which includes both client confrontation and prescription (Heron, 1986). However, Heron argues that, within his analysis, 'catalytic' interventions (those that most nearly match client-centred skills) form the 'bedrock' of good counselling. In this way, Heron seems to endorse the client-centred approach as a basis for effective counselling. Generally, a review of the literature on counselling supports a client-centred basis for practice.

Interestingly, one of the reasons that the approach flourished in the health professions may have been its *simplicity*. Rogers is reported as training many thousands of ex-services personnel in the use of the client-centred approach after the Second World War and in a very short space of time (Kirschenbaum, 1979). Perhaps the fact that it is relatively easy to train health professionals in client-centred counselling, coupled with its positive and life-asserting philosophy, has meant that many trainers have found it an agreeable and acceptable form of communications training. Perhaps, though, we need to seek further and look not just for the relatively easy path to communication but for one which satisfies the individual's needs – and that will never be found within one particular philosophy of counselling. For in adopting the client-centred approach to counselling and care we are, by default, forcing our own world-view on the other person. And here lies the greatest paradox. Ironically, in seeking not to force views on the client, the client-centred counsellor is doing just that by practising the client-centred approach. For, in the end, the client has no option but to accept the style of counselling offered to them.

We might argue, at this point, that the counsellor may declare their interest in the client-centred approach 'up front', at the beginning of the counselling relationship. However, this does not solve the problem. First, the client may be in no position to say 'I would prefer another approach to the one you are offering'. Second, the client may not appreciate that other sorts of counselling are available. Presumably, too, the counsellor who practises client-centred counselling is unlikely to change their orientation when presented with a client who asks for a more prescriptive approach. And herein lies the final problem. The person who practises client-centred counselling is likely to 'believe' in it. They are likely to have been persuaded that this is the appropriate way to counsel people. The more the counsellor practises this type of counselling, the more becomes invested in continuing to do so. The fact remains, however, that there is almost no empirical evidence that *any* sort of counselling 'works'.

In the end it would seem that different approaches to counselling assist different people. Some seem likely to benefit from the client-centred approach while others benefit from more prescriptive approaches. If this is the case (and clearly the case can easily be stated too strongly – it remains supposition) then it follows that the counsellor who offers the greatest range and flexibility of approaches is likely to be of most value overall. On the other hand and in the longer term, it remains vital that we explore exactly what does help other people. We need more research into the helping process and, perhaps, less theory. If health professionals are to continue to use counselling it would be useful to investigate the degree to which it does or does not benefit the people with whom it is used.

What are the implications of this approach for the health professions? First, health professionals in clinical and community practice might feel reassured that they can give information to clients about personal and emotional issues although, oddly, the tendency to overdo this would have to be checked. They might be advised, too, to offer such information *tentatively*, along the lines of 'an approach you may want to think about is …'. All information offered in counselling would have to be up to date and, hopefully, based on research or sound theory. Interestingly enough, this may have the effect of ensuring that all health professionals keep up to date with the knowledge base of their particular field.

Second, there are training implications. Most students are offered training in interpersonal skills and the approach advocated here might widen the possibilities open to trainers. On the other hand, of course, many might reasonably claim that they already use a broad approach. The evidence, however, seems to suggest that the client-centred approach is a popular one, so a variety of other training possibilities might emerge.

Third, there are personal implications for health professionals who have a tendency to use the client-centred approach. Arguably, any position that we hold strongly in relation to our work needs revision on a regular basis. It may be time, then, for those who practise the client-centred approach to take a long hard look at the theoretical and practical implications of the work that they do. This need not mean that all the positive points about the client-centred approach are lost but merely that a synthesis of approaches to counselling may be appropriate.

BASIC COUNSELLING SKILLS

Certain basic counselling skills may be identified although, as we have noted, it is the total relationship that is important, as is the question of meaning. Skills exercised in isolation amount to little: the warmth, genuineness and positive regard must also be present. On the other hand, if basic skills are not considered, then the counselling process will probably be shapeless or it will degenerate into the health-care professional becoming prescriptive. The skill of standing back and allowing the client to find their own way is a difficult one to learn. The following skills may help in the process.

- Questions
- Reflection
- Selective reflection
- Empathy building
- Checking for understanding

Each skill can be learned. In order for that to happen, each must be tried and practised. There is a temptation to say 'I do that anyway!'. The point is to notice the doing of them and to practise doing them better! Whilst counselling often shares the characteristics of everyday conversation, to progress beyond that it is important that some, if not all, of the following skills are used effectively.

Questions

Two main types of questions may be identified in counselling: closed and open questions. A closed question is one that elicits a 'yes', 'no' or similar one-word answer. Or it is one where the questioner can anticipate an approximation of the answer, as she asks it. Examples of closed questions are as follows.

- What is your name?
- How many children do you have?
- Are you happier now?
- Are you still depressed?

Too many closed questions can make the counselling relationship seem like an interrogation! They also inhibit the client's telling of his story and place the locus of responsibility in the relationship firmly with the client. Consider, for instance, the following exchange between marriage guidance counsellor and client:

Counsellor: Are you happier now ... at home?
Client: Yes, I think I am ...
Counsellor: Is that because you can talk more easily with your wife?
Client: I think so ... we seem to get on better, generally.
Counsellor: And has your wife noticed the difference?
Client: Yes, she has.

In this conversation, made up only of closed questions, the counsellor clearly 'leads' the conversation. She also tends to try to influence the client towards accepting the idea that he is 'happier now' and that his wife has 'noticed the difference'. One of the problems with this sort of questioning is that it gives little opportunity for the client to profoundly disagree with the counsellor. In the above exchange, for example, could the client easily have disagreed with the counsellor? It would seem not.

On the other hand, the closed question is useful in clarifying certain specific issues. For example, one may be used as follows.

Client: It's not always easy at home ... the children always seem to be so noisy ... and my wife finds it difficult to cope with them ...
Counsellor: How many children have you?
Client: Three. They're all under ten and they're at the sort of age when they use up a lot of energy and make a lot of noise ...

Here, the closed question is fairly unobtrusive and serves to clarify the conversation. Notice, too, that once the question has been asked, the counsellor allows the client to continue to talk about his family, without further interruption.

Open questions

Open questions are those that do not elicit a particular answer: the health-care professional cannot easily anticipate what an answer will 'look like'. Examples of open questions include:

- What did you do then?
- How did you feel when that happened?
- How are you feeling right now?
- What do you think will happen?

Open questions encourage the client to say more, to expand on their story or to go deeper. An example of their use is as follows.

Counsellor: What is happening at home at the moment?
Client: Things are going quite well. Everyone's much more settled now and my son's found himself a job. He's been out of work for a long time ...

Counsellor: How have you felt about that?
Client: It's upset me a lot … It seemed wrong that I was working and he wasn't … he had to struggle for a long time … he wasn't happy at all …'
Counsellor: And how are you feeling right now?
Client: Upset … I'm still upset … I still feel that I didn't help him enough …

In this conversation, the health-care professional uses only open questions and the client expands on what he thinks and feels. More importantly, perhaps, the above example illustrates the health-care professional 'following' the client and noting his paralinguistic and non-verbal cues. In this way, she is able to help him to focus more on what is happening in the present.

In counselling, open questions are generally preferable to closed ones. They encourage longer, more expansive answers and are rather more free of value judgements and interpretation than are closed questions. All the same, the health-care professional has to monitor the 'slope' of intervention when using open questions. It is easy, for example, to become intrusive by asking too piercing questions, too quickly. As with all counselling interventions, the timing of the use of questions is vital.

When to use questions

Questions can be used in the counselling relationship for a variety of purposes. The main ones include:

- Exploration: 'What else happened …?', 'How did you feel then?'
- For further information: 'How many children have you got?', 'What sort of work were you doing before you retired?'
- To clarify: 'I'm sorry, did you say you want to move or did you say you're not sure?', 'What did you say then …?'
- Encouraging client talk: 'Can you say more about that?', 'What are your feelings about that?'

Other sorts of questions

There are other ways of classifying questions and some to be avoided! Examples of other sorts of questions include:

Leading questions

These are questions that contain an assumption which places the client in an untenable position. The classic example of a leading question is: 'Have you stopped beating your wife?'! Clearly, however the question is answered, the client is in the wrong! Other examples of leading questions are:

- Is your depression the thing that's making your work so difficult?
- Are your family upset by your behaviour?

- Do you think that you may be hiding something ... even from yourself?

The pseudo-analytical questions are particularly awkward. What could the answer possibly be?

Value-laden questions
Questions such as 'Does your homosexuality make you feel guilty' not only pose a moral question but guarantee that the client feels difficult answering them!

'Why' questions
These have been discussed in Chapter 3 and the problems caused by them in the counselling relationship suggest that they should be used very sparingly, if at all.

Confronting questions
Examples of these may include: 'Can you give me an example of when that happened?, and 'Do you still love your wife?'. Confrontation in counselling is quite appropriate once the relationship has fully developed but needs to be used skilfully and appropriately. It is easy for apparent 'confrontation' to degenerate into moralizing. Heron (1986) and Schulman (1982) offer useful approaches to effective confrontation in counselling.

Funnelling

Funnelling (Kahn and Cannell, 1957) refers to the use of questions to guide the conversation from the general to the specific. Thus, the conversation starts with broad, opening questions and slowly, more specific questions are used to focus the discussion. An example of the use of funnelling is as follows.

> **Counsellor**: You seem upset at the moment, what's happening?
> **Client**: It's home ... things aren't working out ...
> **Counsellor**: What's happening at home?
> **Client**: I'm always falling out with Sarah and the children ...
> **Counsellor**: What does Sarah feel about what's happening?
> **Client**: She's angry with me..
> **Counsellor**: About something in particular?
> **Client**: Yes, about the way I talk to Darren, my son ...
> **Counsellor**: What is the problem with Darren?

In this way, the conversation becomes directed and focused and this may pose a problem. If the health-care professional does use funnelling in this way, it is arguable that the counselling conversation is no longer client centred but counsellor directed. In many situations, particularly where shortage of time is an issue, a combination of following and leading may be appropriate. Following refers to the health-care professional taking the lead from the client and exploring the avenues that he wants to explore. Leading refers to the health-care professional taking a more active role and pursuing certain issues that she feels are important. If in doubt, however, the following approach is preferable as it keeps the locus of control in the counselling relationship firmly with the client.

Reflection

Reflection (sometimes called 'echoing') is the process of reflecting back the last few words, or a paraphrase of the last few words, that the client has used in order to encourage them to say more. It is as though the health-care professional is echoing the client's thoughts and that echo serves as a prompt. It is important that the reflection does not turn into a question and this is best achieved by the health-care professional making the repetition in much the same tone of voice as the client used. An example of the use of reflection is as follows.

> **Client**: We had lived in the south for a number of years. Then we moved and I suppose that's when things started to go wrong ...
> **Counsellor**: Things started to go wrong ...
> **Client**: Well, we never really settled down. My wife missed her friends and I suppose I did really ... though neither of us said anything ...
> **Counsellor**: Neither of you said that you missed your friends ...
> **Client**: We both tried to protect each other, really. I suppose if either of us had said anything, we would have felt that we were letting the other one down ...

In this example, the reflections are unobtrusive and unnoticed by the client. They serve to help the client to say more, to develop his story. Used skilfully and with good timing, reflection can be an important method of helping the client. On the other hand, if it is overused or used clumsily, it can appear stilted and is very noticeable. Unfortunately, it is an intervention that takes some practice and one that many people anticipate learning on counselling courses. As a result, when people return from counselling courses, their friends and relatives are often waiting for them to use the technique and may comment on the fact! This should not be a deterrent as the method remains a useful and therapeutic one.

Selective reflection

Selective reflection refers to the method of repeating back to the client a part of something they said that was emphasized in some way or which seemed to be emotionally charged. Thus selective reflection draws from the middle of the client's utterance and not from the end. An example of the use of selective reflection is as follows.

> **Client**: We had just got married. I was very young and I thought things would work out OK. We started buying our own house. My wife hated the place! It was important, though ... we had to start somewhere ...

Counsellor: Your wife hated the house ...

Client: She thought it was the worst place she'd lived in! She reckoned that she would only live there for a year at the most and we ended up being there for five years!

The use of selective reflection allowed the client in this example to develop further an almost throwaway remark. Often, these 'asides' are the substance of very important feelings and the health-care professional can often help in the release of these feelings by using selective reflection to focus on them. Clearly concentration is important, in order to note the points on which to selectively reflect. Also, the counselling relationship is a flowing, evolving conversation which tends to be 'seamless'. Thus the health-care professional should not store up a point which she feels it would be useful to selectively reflect! By the time a break comes in the conversation, the item will probably be irrelevant.

This points up, again, the need to develop 'free-floating attention': the ability to allow the ebb and flow of the conversation to go where the client takes it and for the health-care professional to trust her own ability to choose an appropriate intervention when a break occurs.

Empathy building

This refers to the health-care professional making statements to the client that indicate that she has understood the feeling he is experiencing. A certain intuitive ability is needed here, for often empathy-building statements refer more to what is implied than what is overtly said. An example of the use of empathy-building statements is as follows.

Client: People at work are the same. They're all tied up with their own friends and families ... they don't have a lot of time for me ... though they're friendly enough ...

Counsellor: You sound angry with them ...

Client: I suppose I am! Why don't they take a bit of time to ask me how I'm getting on? It wouldn't take much!

Counsellor: It sounds as though you are saying that people haven't had time for you for a long time ...

Client: They haven't. My family didn't bother much ... I mean, they looked as though they did ... but they didn't really ...

The empathy-building statements used here read between the lines. Now, sometimes such attempts can be completely wrong and the empathy-building statement is rejected by the client. When this happens, it is important for the health-care professional to drop the approach altogether and to pay more attention to listening. Inaccurate empathy-building statements often indicate an eagerness on the part of the health-care professional to become 'involved' with the client's perceptual world at the expense of accurate empathy! Used skilfully, however, they help the client to disclose further and indicate to the client that they are understood.

Checking for understanding

Checking for understanding involves either asking the client if you have understood them correctly or occasionally summarizing the conversation in order to clarify what has been said. The first type of checking is useful when the client quickly covers a lot of topics and seems to be 'thinking aloud'. It can be used to further focus the conversation or as a means of ensuring that you really stay with what the client is saying. The second type of checking should be used sparingly or the counselling conversation can begin to feel rather mechanical and studied. The following two examples illustrate the two uses of checking for understanding.

Example 1

> **Client**: I feel all over the place at the moment ... things aren't quite right at work ... money is still a problem and I don't seem to be talking to anyone ... I'm not sure about work ... sometimes I feel like packing it in ... at other times I think I'm doing OK ...
> **Counsellor**: Let me just clarify ... you're saying things are generally a problem at the moment and you've thought about leaving work?
> **Client**: Yes ... I don't think I will stop work but if I can get to talk it over with my boss, I think I will feel easier about it.

Example 2

> **Counsellor**: Let me see if I can just sum up what we've talked about this afternoon. We mentioned the financial problems and the question of talking to the bank manager. You suggested that you may ask him for a loan. Then you went on to say how you felt you could organize your finances better in the future ...?
> **Client**: Yes, I think that covers most things ...

Some health-care professionals prefer to use the second type of checking at the end of each counselling session and this may help to clarify things before the client leaves. On the other hand, there is much to be said for not 'tidying up' the end of the session in this way. If the loose ends are left, the client continues to think about all the issues that have been discussed as he walks away from the session. If everything is summarized too neatly, the client may feel that the problems can be 'closed down' for a while or, even worse, that they have been 'solved'! Personal problems are rarely simple enough to be summarized in a few words and checking at the end of a session should be used sparingly.

These, then, are particular skills that encourage self-direction on the part of the client and can be learned and used by the health-care professional. They form the basis of all good counselling and can always be returned to as a primary way of working with the client in the counselling relationship.

Helping with emotions

A considerable part of helping people in counselling is concerned with the emotional or 'feelings' side of the person. In the British and North American cultures, a great premium is placed on the individual's being able to 'control' feelings and thus overt expression of emotion is often frowned upon. As a result, we learn to bottle up feelings, sometimes from a very early age. In this chapter, we will consider the effects of such suppression of feelings and identify some practical ways of helping people to identify and explore their feelings.

Types of emotion

Heron (1977) distinguishes between at least four types of emotion that are commonly suppressed or bottled up: anger, fear, grief and embarrassment. He notes a relationship between these feelings and certain overt expressions of them. Thus, in counselling, anger may be expressed as loud sound, fear as trembling, grief through tears and embarrassment by laughter. He notes, also, a relationship between those feelings and certain basic human needs. Heron argues that we all have the need to understand and know what is happening to us. If that knowledge is not forthcoming, we may experience fear. We need to make choices in our lives and if that choice is restricted in certain ways, we may feel anger. We need to experience the expression of love and of being loved. If that love is denied us or taken away from us, we may experience grief. To Heron's basic human needs may be added the need for self-respect and dignity. If such dignity is denied us, we may feel self-conscious and embarrassed. Practical examples of how these relationships 'work' in everyday life and in the counselling relationship may be illustrated as follows.

A 20-year-old girl is attempting to live in a flat on her own. Her parents, however, insist on visiting her regularly and making suggestions as to how she should decorate the flat. They also regularly buy her articles for it and gradually she senses that she is feeling very uncomfortable and distanced from her parents. In the counselling relationship she discovers that she is very angry: her desire to make choices for herself is continually being eroded by her parents' benevolence.

A 48-year-old man hears that his mother is seriously ill and subsequently, she dies. He feels no emotions except that of feeling 'frozen' and unemotional. During a counselling session he suddenly feels the need to cry bitterly. As he does so, he realizes that, many years ago, he had decided that crying was not a masculine thing to do. As a result, he blocked off his grief and felt numb until, within the safety of the counselling relationship, he was able to discover his grief and express it.

A 17-year-old boy, discussing his college work during a counselling session, begins to laugh almost uncontrollably. As he does so, he begins to feel the laughter turning to tears. Through his mixed laughter and tears he acknowledges that 'No one ever took me seriously ... not at school, at home ... or anywhere'. His laughter may be an expression of his lack of self-esteem and his tears, the grief he experiences at that lack.

In the last example it may be noted how emotions that are suppressed are rarely only of one sort. Very often, bottled-up emotion is a mixture of anger, fear, embarrassment and grief. Often, too, the causes of such blocked emotion are unclear and lost in the history of the person. It is perhaps more important that the expression of pent-up emotion is often helpful in that it seems to allow the person to be clearer in his thinking once he has expressed it. It is as though the blocked emotion 'gets in the way' and its release acts as a means of helping the person to clarify his thoughts and feelings. It is notable that the suppression of feelings can lead to certain problems in living that may be clearly identified.

Physical discomfort and muscular pain

Wilhelm Reich, a psychoanalyst with a particular interest in the relationship between emotions and the musculature, noted that blocked emotions could become trapped in the body's muscle clusters (Reich, 1949). Thus he discovered that anger was frequently 'trapped' in the muscles of the shoulders, grief in muscles surrounding the stomach and fear in the leg muscles. Often, these trapped emotions lead to chronic postural problems and the thorough release of the blocked emotion can lead to a freeing up of the muscles and an improved physical appearance. Reich believed in working directly on the muscle clusters in order to bring about emotional release and subsequent freedom from suppression and out of his work was developed a particular type of mind/body therapy, known as 'bioenergetics' (Lowen, 1967; Lowen and Lowen, 1977).

In terms of everyday counselling, trapped emotion is sometimes 'visible' in the way that the client holds himself and the skilled counsellor can learn to notice tension in the musculature and changes in breathing patterns that may suggest muscular tension. We have noted throughout this book how difficult it is to interpret another person's behaviour. What is important here is that such bodily manifestations are only a clue to what may be happening in the person. We cannot assume that a person who looks tense is tense, until he has said that he is.

Health professionals will be very familiar with the link between body posture, the musculature and the emotional state of the person. Frequently, if patients and clients can be helped to relax, then their medical and psychological condition may improve more quickly. Those health professionals who deal most directly with the muscle clusters (remedial gymnasts and physiotherapists, for example) will tend to notice physical tension more readily but all carers can train themselves to observe these important indicators of the emotional status of the person in their care.

Difficulty in decision making

This is a frequent side effect of bottled-up emotion. It is as though the emotion makes the person uneasy and that uneasiness leads to lack of confidence. As a result, the person finds it difficult to rely on his own resources and may find decision making difficult. When we are under stress of any sort, we often feel the need to check decisions with other people. Once some of this stress is removed by talking through problems or by releasing pent-up emotions, the decision-making process often becomes easier.

Faulty self-image

When we bottle up feelings, they often have an unpleasant habit of turning against us. Thus, instead of expressing anger towards others, we turn it against ourselves and feel depressed as a result. Or if we have hung onto unexpressed grief, we turn that grief in on ourselves and experience ourselves as less than we are. Often in counselling, as old resentments or dissatisfactions are expressed, so the person begins to feel better about himself.

Setting unrealistic goals

Tension can lead to further tension which can lead us to set ourselves unreachable targets. It is almost as though we set ourselves up to fail! Sometimes, too, failing is a way of punishing ourselves or it is 'safer' than achieving. Release of tension through the expression of emotion can sometimes help a person to take a more realistic view of himself and his goal setting.

The development of long-term faulty beliefs

Sometimes, emotion that has been bottled up for a long time can lead to a person's view of the world being coloured in a particular way. He learns that 'people can't be trusted' or 'people always let you down in the end'. It is as though old, painful feelings lead to distortions that become part of that person's world-view. Such long-term distorted beliefs about the world do not change easily but may be modified as the person releases feelings and learns to handle his emotions more effectively.

The 'last straw' syndrome

Sometimes, if emotion is bottled up for a considerable amount of time, a valve blows and the person hits out, either literally or verbally. We have all experienced the problem of storing up anger and taking it out on someone else, a process that is sometimes called 'displacement'. The original object of our anger is now replaced by something or someone else. Again, talking through difficulties or the release of pent-up emotion can often help to ensure that the person does not feel the need to explode in this way.

Clearly, no two people react to the bottling up of emotion in the same way. Some people, too, choose not to deal with life events emotionally. It would be curious to argue that there is a 'norm' where emotions are concerned. On the other hand, many people complain of being unable to cope with emotions and if the client feels there is a problem in the emotional domain, then that perception may be expressed as a desire to explore his emotional status.

It is important, however, that the counsellor does not force her particular set of beliefs about feelings and emotions on the client, but waits to be asked to help. Often the request for such help is tacit; the client talks about difficulty in dealing with emotion and that, in itself, may safely be taken as a request for help. A variety of methods is available to the counsellor to help in the exploration of the domain of feelings. Sometimes, these methods produce catharsis, the expression of strong emotion: tears, anger, fear, laughter. Drawing on the literature on the subject, the following statements may be made about the handling of such emotional release.

- Emotional release is usually self-limiting. If the person is allowed to cry or get angry, that emotion will be expressed and then gradually subside. The supportive counsellor will allow it to happen and not become unduly distressed by it.
- Physical support can sometimes be helpful in the form of holding the person's hand or putting an arm round them. Care should be taken, however, that such actions are unambiguous and that the holding is not too 'tight'. A very tight embrace is likely to inhibit the release of emotion. It is worth remembering, also, that not everyone likes or wants physical contact. It is important that the counsellor's support is not seen as intrusive by the client.
- Once the person has had a cathartic release they will need time to piece together the insights that they gain from it. Often all that is needed is for the counsellor to sit quietly with the client while he occasionally verbalizes what he is thinking. The postcathartic period can be a very important stage in the counselling process.
- There seems to be a link between the extent to which we can 'allow' another person to express emotion and the degree to which we can handle our own emotion. This is another reason why the counsellor needs self-awareness. To help others explore their feelings we need, first, to explore our own. Many colleges and university departments offer workshops on cathartic work and self-awareness development that can aid the counsellor in both helping others and gaining self-insight.
- Frequent 'cathartic counselling' can be exhausting for the counsellor and if she is to avoid burnout, she needs to set up a network of support from other colleagues or via a peer support group. We cannot expect to constantly handle other people's emotional release without its taking a toll on us.

Methods of helping the client to explore feelings

These are practical methods that can be used in the counselling relationship to help the client identify, examine and, if required, release emotion. Most of them will be more effective if the counsellor has first tried them on herself. This can be done simply by reading through the description of them and then trying them out, in your mind. Alternatively, they can be tried out with a colleague or friend. Another way of exploring their effectiveness is to use them in a peer support context. The setting up and running of such a group is described in the next chapter, along with various exercises that can be used to improve counselling skills. All the following activities should be used gently and thoughtfully and timed to fit in with the client's requirements. There should never be any sense of pushing the client to explore feelings because of a misplaced belief that 'a good cry will do him good!'.

Giving permission

Sometimes in counselling, the client tries desperately to hang on to strong feelings and not to express them. As we have seen, this may be due to the cultural norm which suggests that holding on is better than letting go. Thus a primary method for helping someone to explore his emotions is for the counsellor to 'give permission' for the expression of feeling. This can be done simply through acknowledging that 'It's all right with me if you feel you are going to cry …'. In this way the counsellor has reassured the client that expression of feelings is acceptable within the relationship. Clearly, a degree of tact is required here. It is important that the client does not feel pushed into expressing feelings that he would rather not express. The 'permission giving' should never be coercive nor should there be an implicit suggestion that 'you must express your feelings!'.

Literal description

This refers to inviting the client to go back in his memory to a place that he is, currently, only alluding to and describe that place in some detail. An example of this use of literal description is as follows.

> **Client**: I used to get like this at home … I used to get very upset …
> **Counsellor**: Just go back home for a moment … describe one of the rooms in the house …
> **Client**: The front room faces directly out onto the street … there is an armchair by the window … the TV in the corner … our dog is lying on the rug … it's very quiet …
> **Counsellor**: What are your feeling right now?
> **Client**: Like I was then … angry … upset …

Describing in literal terms a place that was the scene of an emotional experience can often bring that emotion back. It is important that the description has an 'I am there' quality about it and does not slip into a detached description, such as: 'We lived in a big house which wasn't particularly modern but then my parents didn't like modern houses much ...'.

Locating and developing a feeling in terms of the body
As we have noted above, very often feelings are accompanied by a physical sensation. It is often helpful to identify that physical experience and to invite the client to exaggerate it, to allow the feeling to 'expand' in order to explore it further. Thus, an example of this approach is as follows.

> **Counsellor**: How are you feeling at the moment?
> **Client**: Slightly anxious.
> **Counsellor**: Where, in terms of your body, do you feel the anxiety?
> **Client**: (rubs stomach) Here.
> **Counsellor**: Can you increase that feeling in your stomach?
> **Client**: Yes, it's spreading up to my chest.
> **Counsellor**: And what's happening now?
> **Client**: It reminds me of a long time ago ... when I first started work ...
> **Counsellor**: What happened there ...?

Again, the original suggestion by the counsellor is followed by a question to elicit how the client is feeling. This gives the client a chance to identify the thoughts that go with the feeling and to explore them further.

Empty chair
In this method the counsellor invites the client to imagine the feeling that they are experiencing as 'sitting' in a chair opposite them and then have them address the feeling. This can be used in a variety of ways and the next examples show its applications.

> **Client**: I feel very confused at the moment, I can't seem to sort things out ...
> **Counsellor**: Can you imagine your confusion sitting in that chair over there ... what does it look like?
> **Client**: It looks like a great big ball of wool ... how odd!
> **Counsellor**: If you could speak to your confusion, what would you say to it?
> **Client**: I wish I could sort you out!
> **Counsellor**: And what's your confusion saying back to you?
> **Client**: I'm glad you don't sort me out – I stop you from having to make any decisions!
> **Counsellor**: And what do you make of that?
> **Client**: I suppose that could be true ... the longer I stay confused, the less I have to make decisions about my family ...

> **Counsellor**: How are you feeling about the people you work with ... you said you found it quite difficult to get on with them ...
> **Client**: Yes, it's still difficult, especially my boss.

Counsellor: Imagine your boss is sitting in that chair over there ... how does that feel?
Client: Uncomfortable! He's angry with me!
Counsellor: What would you like to say to him?
Client: Why do I always feel scared of you ... why do you make me feel uncomfortable?
Counsellor: And what does he say?
Client: I don't! It's you that feels uncomfortable, not me ... You make yourself uncomfortable ... (to the counsellor) He's right! I do make myself uncomfortable but I use him as an excuse ...

The empty chair can be used in a variety of ways to set up a dialogue between either the client and his feelings or between the client and a person that the client talks 'about'. It offers a very direct way of exploring relationships and feelings and deals directly with the issue of 'projection', the tendency we have to see qualities in others that are, in fact, our own. Using the empty chair technique can bring to light those projections and allow the client to see them for what they are. Other applications of this method are described in detail by Perls (1969).

Contradiction
It is sometimes helpful if the client is asked to contradict a statement that they make, especially when that statement contains some ambiguity. An example of this approach is as follows.

Client: (looking at the floor) I've sorted everything out now: everything's OK.
Counsellor: Try contradicting what you've just said ...
Client: Everything's not OK ... Everything isn't sorted out' ... (laughs) ... That's true, of course ... there's a lot more to sort out yet ...

Mobilization of body energy
Developing the idea that emotions can be trapped within the body's musculature, it is sometimes helpful for the counsellor to suggest to the client that he stretches or takes some very deep breaths. In the process, the client may become aware of tensions that are trapped in his body and begin to recognize and identify those tensions. This, in turn, can lead to the client talking about and expressing some of those tensions. This is particularly helpful if, during the counselling conversation, the client becomes less and less 'mobile' and adopts a particularly hunched or curled-up position in his chair. The invitation to stretch serves almost as a contradiction to the body position being adopted by the client at that time.

Exploring fantasy
We often set fairly arbitrary limits on what we think we can and cannot do. When a client seems to be doing this, it is sometimes helpful to explore what may happen if this limit was broken. An example of this is as follows.

Client: I'd like to be able to go abroad for a change, I never seem to go very far on holiday.

Counsellor: What stops you?

Client: Flying, I suppose …

Counsellor: What's the worst thing about flying?

Client: I get very anxious.

Counsellor: And what happens if you get very anxious?

Client: Nothing really! I just get anxious!

Counsellor: So nothing terrible will happen if you allow yourself to get anxious?

Client: No, not really … I hadn't thought about it like that before …

Rehearsal

Sometimes the anticipation of a coming event or situation provokes anxiety. The counsellor can help the client to explore a range of feelings by rehearsing a future event with him. Thus if the client is anticipating a forthcoming interview, the counsellor could act the role of interviewer, with a discussion afterwards. The client who wants to develop the assertive behaviour to enable him to challenge his boss may benefit from role playing the situation in the counselling session. In each case, it is important that both client and counsellor 'get into role' and that the session does not just become a discussion of what may or may not happen. The actual playing through and rehearsal of a situation is nearly always more powerful than a discussion of it.

Alberti and Emmons (1982) offer some suggestions about how to set up role plays and exercises for developing assertive behaviour and Wilkinson and Canter (1982) describe some approaches to developing socially skilled behaviour. Often, if the client can practise effective behaviour, then the appropriate thoughts and feelings can accompany that behaviour. The novelist Kurt Vonnegut wryly commented that: 'We are what we pretend to be – so take care what you pretend to be' (Vonnegut, 1969). Sometimes, the first stage in changing is trying out a new pattern of behaviour or a new way of thinking and feeling. Practice, therefore, is invaluable.

This approach develops from the idea that what we think influences what we feel and do. If our thinking is restrictive, we may begin to feel that we can or cannot do certain things. Sometimes having these barriers to feeling and doing challenged can free a person to think, feel and act differently.

The domain of feelings is frequently addressed in counselling. Counselling people who want to explore feelings takes time and cannot be rushed. Also, the development and use of the various skills described here is not the whole of the issue. Health professionals working with emotions need, also, to have developed warmth, genuineness, empathic understanding and unconditional positive regard. Emotional counselling can never be a mechanical process as it is one that touches the lives of both client and counsellor.

COUNSELLING AS CONFESSION

One of the features of counselling is that it allows clients to tell counsellors things that they may not have told other people. In a sense, then, there is a *confessional* element to counselling. We can say things to counsellors and not get rebuffed or judged as a result. This leads to a sense of being accepted, something that is reinforced in the literature. Acceptance seems to be an important part of what counsellors do with clients. It does, of course, raise the question of how far counsellors can accept what the client says as 'acceptable'. Can we ask the counsellor to accept *everything* that the client says? Or should the counsellor feel entitled to show surprise, indignation or even lack of acceptance of what they hear? This must remain an open question. One of the apparent contradictions in the Rogerian approach to counselling is that Rogers calls for both acceptance *and* genuineness. It may be that these two are, in certain circumstances, incompatible. If I find it difficult to accept what another person is telling me, is it 'genuine' to appear to accept what I hear or should I (through 'genuineness') comment on the fact that what I am hearing is difficult to accept? Should the counsellor be a sponge who offers a neutral value position or can they offer a personal opinion on what the client is saying? Again, these questions must remain open. As with most aspects of counselling, there are no hard and fast rules about what is or what is not 'right'.

COUNSELLING AS VOYEURISM

This is the other side of the 'confessional' coin. It seems possible that counsellors may act as voyeurs in relation to some of their clients. We are, perhaps, all fairly nosy. We like to know what other people are up to. The counsellor must always be alert to the possibility that they are *enjoying* listening to a particular story that the client is telling. If this happens, it seems quite possible that the counsellor will encourage the client to elaborate on a particular aspect of their story. In this case, the counsellor is working at fulfilling their own needs rather than those of the client.

A FORMAT FOR ORGANIZING COUNSELLING

Not all of the issues discussed by a client are of equal importance. The health professional often has to assess situations quickly and 'counselling' may take place in less than ideal circumstances. It seems reasonable, then, to offer a format for considering *priorities* in counselling and this is given in Figure 5.1.

Immediate health issues	Is the client's immediate health cause for concern. Should any medical intervention be made immediately. If so, should the client be 'referred on'?
Safety issues	Is the client safe in terms of their housing, accommodation, home situation? Is mortgage/rent being paid? Is the physical environment in which the client lives a cause for immediate concern? If so, what needs to be done?
Psychological issues	What is your assessment of the client's mood? Do they talk about depression, anxiety or other signs of psychological distress? If so, is further treatment warranted?
Longer term health issues	What is the general status of the client's health? Are they receiving long-term medication for conditions such as hypertension, diabetes or other long-standing illness? Is such medication being taken?
Personal goals and aims	What does the client identify as their immediate and longer term needs and wants?

Figure 5.1   Priorities in counselling.

SUMMARY

Counselling skills are a basic prerequisite for any effective health-care professional. The skills discussed in this chapter are applicable in a wide range of health-care settings. This chapter has also considered what counselling might be, the problems associated with it and has taken a critical look at the issue of client-centred counselling.

References

Alberti, R.E. and Emmons, M.L. (1982) *Your Perfect Right: A Guide to Assertive Living*, Impact, San Luis Obispo, California.

Allcock, N. (1992) Teaching the skills of assessment through the use of an experiential workshop. *Nurse Education Today*, **12**(4), 287–92.

Aptekar, H.H. (1955) *The Dynamics of Casework and Counselling*, Houghton Mifflin, Cambridge, Mass.

Breese, J. (1983) Counselling pupils in centres for disruptives. *Maladjustment and Therapeutic Education*, **1**(1), 6–12.

British Association for Counselling (BAC) (1984) *Code of Ethics and Practice for Counsellors*, BAC, Rugby.

British Association for Counselling (BAC) (1989) *Invitation to Membership*, BAC, Rugby.

Burks, H.M. and Stefflre, D. (1979) *Theories of Counselling*, 3rd edn, McGraw-Hill, New York.

Burnard, P. (1989) *Counselling Skills for Health Professionals*, Chapman & Hall, London.

Burnard, P. (1992) *Experiential Learning in Action*, Avebury, Aldershot.

Burnard, P. (1995) *Learning Human Skills: A Reflective and Experiential Guide for Nurses*, 3rd edn, Butterworth-Heinemann, Oxford.

Claxton, G. (1984) *Live and Learn: An Introduction to the Psychology of Growth and Change in Everyday Life*, Harper & Row, London.

English, H.B. and English, A. (1958) *A Comprehensive Dictionary of Psychological and Psychoanalytical Terms*, Longmans, New York.

Heron, J. (1977) *Catharsis in Human Development*, Human Potential Research Project, University of Surrey, Guildford, Surrey.

Heron, J. (1986) *Six Category Intervention Analysis*, 2nd edn, Human Potential Research Project, University of Surrey, Guildford, Surrey.

Kahn, R.L. and Cannell, C.F. (1957) *The Dynamics of Interviewing*, Wiley, New York.

Kelly G. (1955) *The Psychology of Personal Constructs, Vols I and II*, W.W. Norton, New York.

King-Spooner, S. (1995) Psychotherapy and the white dodo. *Changes*, **13**(1), 45–51.

Kirschenbaum, H. (1979) *On Becoming Carl Rogers*, Dell, New York.

Knowles, M. (1975) *Self Directed Learning*, Cambridge Books, New York.

Knowles, M. (1978) *The Adult Learner: A Neglected Species*, 2nd edn, Gulf, Texas.

Kreps, G.L. and Query, J.L. (1990) Health communication and interpersonal competence, in *Speech Communication: Essays to Commemorate the 75th anniversary of The Speech Communication Association* (eds G.M. Phillips and J.T. Woods), Southern Illinois University Press, Carbondale, Illinois.

Lowen, A. (1967) *Betrayal of the Body*, Macmillan, New York.

Lowen, A. and Lowen, L. (1977) *The Way to Vibrant Health: A Manual of Bioenergetic Exercises*, Harper & Row, New York.

Lyotard, J.-F. (1983) Answering the question, What is postmodernism? in *Innovation/Renovation* (eds I. Hassan and S. Hassan), University of Wisconsin Press, Madison, Wisconsin.

Masson, J. (1988) *Against Therapy*, Fontana/Collins, London.

May, R. (1989) Answer to Ken Wilber and John Rowan. *Journal of Humanistic Psychology*, **29**(2), 244–8.

McLeod, J. (1994) *Doing Research in Counselling*, Sage, London.

Murgatroyd, S. (1985) *Counselling and Helping*, Methuen, London.

Nelson-Jones, R. (1995) *The Theory and Practice of Counselling*, Cassell, London.

Nichols, K.A (1991) Counselling and renal failure, in *Counselling and Communication in Health Care* (eds H. David and L. Fallowfield), Wiley, Chichester.

Noonan, E. (1983) *Counselling Young People*, Methuen, London.

Perls, F. (1969) *Gestalt Therapy Verbatim*, Real People Press, Lafayette, California.

Peters, R.S. (1969) *Ethics and Education*, Allen & Unwin, London.

Reich, W. (1949) *Character Analysis*, Simon & Schuster, New York.

Rogers, C.R. (1952) *Client-Centred Therapy*, Constable, London.

Rogers, C.R. (1967) *On Becoming a Person*, Constable, London.

Rogers, C.R. (1983) *Freedom to Learn for the Eighties*, Merril, Columbus, Ohio.

Sartre, J.-P. (1956) *Being and Nothingness*, Philosophical Library, New York.

Sartre, J.-P. (1973) *Humanism and Existentialism*, Methuen, London.

Schulman, E.D. (1982) *Intervention in the Human Services: A Guide to Skills and Knowledge*, 3rd edn, Mosby, St Louis, Missouri.

Vonnegut, K. (1969) *Mother Night*, Gollancz, London.

Wilkinson, J. and Canter, S. (1982) *Social Skills Training Manual: Assessment, Programme Design and Management of Training*, Wiley, Chichester.

Group facilitation skills

AIMS OF THE CHAPTER

The following issues and skills are discussed.

- Types of groups
- Group life
- Group dynamics
- Group facilitation skills

Health-care professionals often need to facilitate groups. To run groups effectively and therapeutically, they have to make certain decisions about how they will run groups. This chapter considers aspects of group facilitation.

First, what sorts of groups are health-care professionals likely to find themselves facilitating? A shortlist would include the following.

- Education groups
- Discussion groups
- Therapy groups
- Relative support groups
- Case conferences
- Curriculum planning groups
- Stress/relaxation groups

Whilst each of these groups has different aims, the skills required to facilitate them are similar. The overall objective will be to enable a group of people to make the best possible use of the time that they have at their disposal. The health-care professional acting as facilitator needs to notice her own style of facilitation and its strengths and deficits. Once those strengths and deficits have become explicit, the strengths can be reinforced and the deficits made good.

A MAP OF THE GROUP PROCESS

Tuckman (1965) offered a useful map of the group process. He noted that every group passes through four stages in its development. He described these as the stages of forming, storming, norming and performing. During the forming stage, group members meet each other for the first time and attempt to discover what behaviour is and is not required of them. This is a time for testing the water, discovering other people and discovering one's role in the group. In many ways, the new member of the group is 'on her best behaviour': the real person has yet to emerge.

In the storming stage, group members begin to thaw out a little. As a result they characteristically become hostile with one another as they battle to assert themselves and to stamp their personalities on the group. This is the stage of conflict between 'my' needs and wants and those of the group. Often this is a painful period in which there are fights for leadership of the group and attempts at establishing a pecking order. Health-care professionals in the early stages of their education and training, for example, may notice the advent of the storming stage once the introductory period in the school or college has been worked through or towards the end of their first year. In this stage, friendships and loyalties are tested and certain individuals may either opt out of the group and leave the education and training course or feel pressurized to leave by the group.

Out of the storming stage develops the norming stage, when the group comes to terms with itself and the individuals in it resolve their conflicts to some degree, both personal and interpersonal. In order for the group to function harmoniously, rules, both written and unwritten, are established in the group's resolve to become more cohesive. Members typically get to know one another better and a more trusting, intimate atmosphere develops. When they reach this stage, courses are often perceived as having established themselves. The group feels as though it has arrived!

The danger here is that such groups will become too settled and too complacent. There is also a problem when groups are too readily socialized into the norms of the institution. In this case, they tend to readily accept what they see and lose a certain critical faculty. It is important that all health-care professionals maintain the ability to think critically and are able to challenge the prevailing practices in the clinical areas in which they work. In most large institutions there develops what has been called an 'organizational culture'. That is to say that institutions, as large groups themselves, develop their own norms and seek to initiate newcomers into those norms in order for things to go along much as they have in the past. The new group not only has to develop its own norms but may find itself in conflict or disagreement with the norms of the organizational culture.

The norming stage leads on to the most productive phase of group life, the performing stage. Here, the group has developed a mature collective identity and members are able to work easily and usefully together. The danger again arises at this stage that the group may become complacent and that new growth is not encouraged.

This can be seen in certain clinical environments where everyone has worked together for a considerable period and people have come to know each other, their habits and behaviours well. Such a group can become inward looking and reject both new ideas and new members. Students joining such groups often feel left out or that they are intruding. The group that arrives at the performing stage needs to keep itself alert to changes and suggestion from outside.

'Groupthink', the term sometimes used to describe the tendency for groups to work as if they were one closed-minded individual, can occur if the group does not remain in touch and awake to other groups and to new ideas. It could be argued that many health professional groups and perhaps the profession itself has a tendency towards such closed thinking.

This then is a typical cycle through which most groups seem to pass. It may be viewed as a lifecycle of the group directly comparable to the lifecycle of the individual; it mimics childhood, adolescence, young adulthood and maturity. Viewed in this light, the group experiences can be valuable for developing further individual awareness. Monitoring personal behaviour and responses in the group can provide insights for individuals through appreciating this correlation between the lifecycle of the group and the lifecycle of the individual.

A member of the group may see herself as 'reliving' stages of her own life when she joins that group. The group is perhaps the most potent medium through which to develop self-awareness. In the group both self-disclosure and feedback from others take place – two vital ingredients for self-awareness.

If the metaphor of the lifecycle of the group is accepted, it will be understood that a group may well reach the point where it has fulfilled its function and the cycle has been completed. In health-care professional education and training this disbanding of the group comes naturally at the end of a three- or four-year period, predetermined by the college, school or examining body. In other groups, however, such a time period may not be so clearcut and it is important that at intervals through any performing period, the group reviews its performance and function. There is little value in continuing when the point of the group's existence has been exhausted. There is nothing worse that belonging to a 'dead' group.

Following from the issue of the group's stages comes the question of the processes that occur during the group's life. All that happens in a group may be divided into two aspects:

1. content
2. processes.

Content refers to all that is talked about in any given group. Processes are all those things that happen in a group: the dynamics of the group. Such processes occur in all groups of all types. They are more noticeable in small, intimate groups but also frequently occur in professional and work groups. They have been so frequently noted that they are easily described.

Recognition of such processes is vital for anyone running groups and it is helpful if group members learn to recognize them. Once again, developing such awareness is part of the larger task of developing personal awareness. It is often useful if the group facilitator holds a discussion about group processes at one of the early meetings of that group. She may also like to invite group members to notice these processes as they occur, so developing a sense of group reflexivity. Time can then be put aside at regular intervals to discuss the perceived processes. In self-awareness groups, discussion of processes is just as important as the discussion of content. It is regrettable that traditional educational methods have mostly concentrated on the content of courses and study periods at the expense of exploring processes.

GROUP PROCESSES

Pairing can be noted when two individuals, usually sitting next to each other, engage in a quiet and often hesitant conversation with each other. The conversation may occur as a series of 'asides', facial expressions and, the extreme form, the passing of notes! Pairing is distracting for other group members and may occur as a result of disaffection with the group, insecurity on the part of one or both of the pair involved, boredom or as a means of testing group leadership. Another form of pairing can be seen when two group members form a fairly exclusive relationship and support each other in a determined manner whenever either of them makes a contribution to group affairs and particularly when either of them is under attack from any other group member.

Projection occurs when an individual identifies the group as being responsible for her feelings. The person sees a quality in the group which is, in fact, a quality of her own but of which she is unaware. Thus the individual may say 'this group is hostile and unfriendly', when it is plain to the rest of the group that such a description fits the group member herself. Such projection may arise out of insecurity in the group or out of the individual's own lack of awareness.

The process of 'owning' projections and taking responsibility for oneself can be a particularly valuable piece of experiential learning in the group. On the other hand, you have to be careful. Not everything that a person says about a group is a projection. Sometimes they are merely describing what is obviously true about the group. So how do you distinguish between a projection and a description? No easy task! Some guidelines that may help here are:

- a projection is usually only experienced by one person;
- the rest of the group usually disagrees with a projection;
- often the individual comes to recognize her own projections, especially if she is on the lookout for them;
- descriptions are usually corroborated by other group members;
- descriptions do not usually have the 'emotional tone' that can accompany projections.

Scapegoating often occurs during the storming stage of the group. The group looks for someone to blame for the way they are feeling and behaving and chooses a fairly quiet or vulnerable member on whom to vent their feelings. In this sense, scapegoating is a type of collective bullying. Alternatively, the group finds an outside scapegoat and blames 'the organization' or 'the profession' for the circumstances in which it finds itself. This is the 'group beef'. Usually this blaming of outside organizations or bodies is a means of the group avoiding responsibility for itself or a way of avoiding making decisions. Recognition of such scapegoating is part of the group leader's role and identification of it by the group itself can lead to a sense of growing cohesion and personal awareness. Again, though, a word of caution. Sometimes the organization or the profession *is* to blame! It is important to make the distinction.

When a group member becomes 'shut down' (Heron, 1973), they cut themselves off from the rest of the group, often feeling swamped by it and emotionally fragile. This may be caused by the group member suddenly identifying with a painful experience being described by someone else. It may be a response to the general emotional tone of the group or a rejection of the ideas being put forward in the group discussion. The skilled group facilitator recognizes such shutting down and helps the individual either to express her feelings or to quietly rejoin the group. There will be occasions, too, when the group member favours a short break from the group. Shutting down often occurs when a group member begins to face important emotional issues that have previously been buried.

The shut-down person is in crisis. She cannot face her feelings and she cannot verbalize how she feels. Working through such a phase must be handled tactfully and sensitively and the person should never be rushed or told that expressing her pent-up feelings would 'do her good'. Sometimes it would, sometimes it wouldn't. The point is that it is the individual's place to decide whether or not now is a good time to work through the bottled-up feelings.

The person who 'rescues' may be a 'compulsive carer'. She may find it easier to defend others from attack than to let those people fend for themselves and learn from the experience. Often rescuing others is a means of avoiding dealing with personal problems: to be seen as the person who always comes to another's aid can serve as a smokescreen for covering unresolved conflicts. It may be that many health-care professionals are compulsive carers. Often it is easier to care for others than it is to care for ourselves. This is fine as far as it goes but constantly caring for and rescuing others is a recipe for burnout and emotional exhaustion.

Part of the process of developing self-awareness includes standing back and enabling others to learn through experience rather than rushing in and helping too quickly. Often the temptation is to protect others from that which we cannot take ourselves. We feel that 'if I can't take it, she can't', forgetting that the other person is a *different* person and blurring the distinction between 'me' and 'you'. As we gain awareness and resilience, we can 'allow' others to live their own life without being overprotected or denied the chance to develop their own coping skills.

This applies to a wide range of health-care situations: the patient who learns to cope with their anxiety develops the ability to cope with it again; the person who is allowed to live through a certain amount of pain develops the ability to deal with pain. If we constantly 'rescue' we constantly deny people the ability to develop autonomy.

Of course there are limits to this. The group facilitator has responsibilities towards the members of her group and some judgements have to be made about the degree of rescuing that she can perform. As a general rule, she may want to 'rescue' members who are being scapegoated in the early days of the group's development. As the group progresses, she can rescue less and less and allow individuals to fend for themselves more and more.

The group process known as flight can be demonstrated in various ways. The group which avoids difficult issues or decisions can be said to be taking flight. The individual group member who is constantly humorous and light-hearted may also be taking flight in humour. The member who always has a theoretical explanation for everything may be taking flight from feelings. Yet another form of flight is keeping group discussion on a superficial level, so that deep and more disturbing issues are kept safely at a distance. Identifying and working through flight is a means of helping the group to grow. Self-disclosure occurs more readily when flight is avoided and group members are able to share each other's experiences on an adult-to-adult basis.

Again, this is not to say that all laughter is flight or that the group should always be deep and profound. It is merely to acknowledge that we all avoid facing ourselves, especially in the company of others.

In looking at group processes, it is worth noting that the energy level of any group will fluctuate from time to time just as an individual's energy level will have its peaks and troughs. Part of the development of group life involves living through the periods of low energy and taking advantage of the peaks. Again, the skilful leader and skilful group member will notice such fluctuations, take responsibility for them and make adjustments as necessary. When group energy does drop, the following courses of action by the facilitator may be appropriate.

- Sit it out and see what happens.
- Suggest a change of activity.
- Draw the group's attention to the drop in energy.
- Take a short break.

CHARACTERISTICS OF ALL GROUPS

Small groups have things in common. Dorothy Stock Whittington (1987) offers a useful list of the characteristics of groups.

1. Groups develop particular moods and atmospheres.

2. Shared themes can build up in groups.
3. Groups evolve norms and belief systems.
4. Groups vary in cohesiveness and in the permeability of their boundaries.
5. Groups develop and change their character over a period of time.
6. Persons occupy different positions in groups with respect to power, centrality and being liked and disliked.
7. Individuals in groups sometimes find one or two other persons who are especially important to them because they are similar in some respect to significant persons in the individual's life or to significant aspects of the self.
8. Social comparison can take place in a group.
9. A group is an environment in which persons can observe what others do and say and then observe what happens next.
10. A group is an environment in which persons can receive feedback from others concerning their own behaviour or participation.

Arguably, these characteristics are true of most small groups, from clinical case conferences to learning groups and from therapy groups to discussion groups. The list offers considerable material for discussion with both peers and students and may be a useful starting point for teaching about groups and group dynamics.

DIMENSIONS OF FACILITATOR STYLE

Heron (1989) offers a sixfold model of facilitator styles. These six aspects of facilitation he calls dimensions. These are different aspects from those presented in Chapter 1. It seems to me that both versions have much to commend them and the two versions can be used in a wide range of therapeutic and educational contexts. The dimensions are as follows.

- The planning dimension
- The meaning dimension
- The confronting dimension
- The feeling dimension
- The structuring dimension
- The valuing dimension

The six dimensions of facilitator style may be used to make decisions about how this group is run at this time. Not all of the dimensions will be used in every group. Decisions about which dimension will be used during which group will depend on the type of group being run, the aims of that group, the personality of the facilitator and the needs of the participants.

The dimensions cover most aspects of the setting up and running of groups. What follows is an adapted version of Heron's model.

The planning dimension

This dimension is concerned with the setting up of the group. Group members always need to know why they are in a particular group. Therefore the group facilitator needs to make certain decisions about how to identify the aims and objectives of the group. She has at least three options here.

1. She can decide upon the aims and objectives herself, before setting up the group at all.
2. She can negotiate the aims and objectives with the group. In this case, she will decide on some of those aims and objectives and the group will decide on others.
3. She can encourage the group to set its own aims and objectives. In this case, all the facilitator does is to turn up on a certain day with a 'title' or name for the group. All further decisions about what the group is to achieve are made by the group.

The first example above illustrates the traditional learning group approach. The educator who uses this approach will have set aims and objectives for a particular lesson, planned in advance.

The second example illustrates the negotiated group approach. The health-care professional working as a group therapist (for example) will meet the group for the first time and work with them to identify what that group can achieve in the time that they meet together.

The third example illustrates the fully client-centred or student-centred approach to working with groups. Here, the health-care professional does not anticipate the needs or wants of the group at all. Instead, she allows the learning, therapy or discussion group to set its own agenda. Such an approach needs careful handling if it is not to degenerate into an aimless series of meetings.

Other aspects of the planning dimension include making decisions about the following issues.

•   The number of group participants.
•   Whether or not particular 'rules' will apply to the group.
•   Whether or not group membership will remain the same throughout the life of the group (the closed group) or whether new members will be allowed to join (the open group).

Again, such planning decisions can be taken either unilaterally by the facilitator or via negotiation with the group.

The meaning dimension

This aspect of group facilitation is concerned with what sense group members make of being in the group. As with the previous dimension, at least three options are open here.

1. The facilitator can offer explanations, theories or models to enable group members to make sense of what is happening. Thus a health-care professional running a support group for bereaved relatives may offer a theoretical model of bereavement to give those relatives a framework for understanding what is happening to them.
2. The facilitator may sometimes offer 'interpretations' of what is going on. At other times, she will listen to group members' perceptions of what is happening. This may frequently happen in an open discussion group or a case conference.
3. The facilitator offers no explanations or theories but encourages group members to verbalize their own ideas, thoughts and theories. This is the non-directive mode of working with meaning in a group.

The confronting dimension

When people work together, all sorts of conflicts can arise. Sometimes these conflicts are overt and show themselves in arguments and disagreements. Sometimes, a 'hidden agenda' is at work. Conflicts sit just beneath the surface of group life. Whilst they affect it in various ways, they cannot be worked with unless the group addresses them directly. The confronting dimension of facilitation is concerned with ways in which individual members and the group as a whole are challenged. The three ways of working in this dimension are as follows.

1. The facilitator can challenge the group or its members directly. Thus, she asks questions, makes suggestions, offers interpretations of behaviour in the group. Her aim is to encourage the group and its members to confront what is happening at various levels.
2. The facilitator can encourage an atmosphere in which people feel safe enough to challenge each other (and the facilitator). In this process, the following 'ground rules' for direct and clear communication can help:

    *   say 'I' rather than 'you', 'we' or 'people' when discussing issues in the group;
    *   speak directly to other people, rather than about them. Thus 'I am angry with you, David' is better than 'I am angry with people in this group'.

3. The facilitator can choose not to confront at all. In this case, two things may happen: no confrontation takes place and the group gets 'stuck' or the group learns to challenge itself, without assistance from the facilitator.

The first example of confrontation above is the traditional 'chairperson' mode of facilitation. The facilitator who uses this approach stays in control of the group. The negotiated style of confrontation can be used in discussion groups and informal teaching sessions. The third example can be used in meetings and discussions of a very formal kind. If it is used in therapy and self-awareness groups, the chances are that either the 'hidden agenda' will not be addressed or the group members will outgrow the need for the facilitator. All groups should aim at becoming independent of the group leader.

The feeling dimension

Therapy groups, self-awareness groups and certain sorts of learning groups tend to generate emotion in participants. The feeling dimension is concerned with how such emotional expression is dealt with. Decisions that can be made in this domain include the following.

• Will emotional release be encouraged? This may be appropriate in a therapy or social skills training group.
• Is there to be an explicit contract with the group about emotional release? Here, the facilitator may suggest at the beginning of the first group meeting that emotional release is 'allowed', thus giving group members permission to express emotions.
• Does the facilitator feel skilled in handling emotional release? If not, she may want to develop skills in coping with other people's feelings, especially when these involve the overt expression of tears, anger or fear. Training in cathartic work is needed here.

The structuring dimension

Structure is a necessary part of group life. Without it, the group can fall apart. The issue here is how such structure is developed. Again, at least three options exist in this domain.

1. The facilitator can decide on the total structure of the group. In a social skills group, for example, she may introduce a variety of exercises and activities that allow participants to learn how to answer the telephone, introduce themselves at parties or take faulty goods back to a shop. At all times, she remains in control of the overall structure.
2. The facilitator can encourage group members to organize certain aspects of the life and structure of the group. Thus the ward sister who is running a learning group may invite students to read and discuss seminar papers. In this respect, she is handing over some of the structure to group members.
3. The facilitator can play a minimal role in structuring the life of the group. The extreme example of this is the Tavistock approach to group therapy in which the only structure is the starting and finishing times. Between those times the facilitator makes no attempt to 'lead' the group. This is not for the uninitiated!

As a general rule it is probably better for the new facilitator to start with lots of structure (which is imposed by her). As she gains confidence in running groups, she can gradually hand over some of that structure to group members.

The valuing dimension

This aspect of group facilitation is concerned with creating a supportive and valuing atmosphere in which the group can work. No group will succeed if the atmosphere is one of distrust ahd suspicion. The issues here are the following.

- Is the facilitator confident enough to allow disagreement, discussion and varieties of points of view?
- Does she have sufficient self-awareness to know the effect that she is having on the group?
- Is she skilled, positive, life asserting and encouraging?

Learning to value other people (and oneself) comes with experience of running groups, developing a range of therapeutic skills such as counselling, social skills and assertiveness.

SUMMARY

Facilitation can be an exhilarating and educational experience for health-care professionals and educators. Most health-care professionals need to become proficient in working with people in groups. The skills involved have wide application within the field of health care, with direct and indirect effects on improving the quality of education, management and care. This chapter has described some of the sorts of decisions that the new facilitator may want to make about how to run clinical, managerial or training groups.

References

Heron, J. (1973) *Experiential Training Techniques*, Human Potential Research Project, University of Surrey, Guildford, Surrey.

Heron, J. (1989) *Facilitators' Manual*, Kogan Page, London.

Tuckman, B. (1965) Developmental sequences in small groups. *Psychological Bulletin*, **63**(6), 384–99.

Whittington, D.S. (1987) *Using Groups To Help People*, Tavistock/Routledge, London.

Skills check: Part Two

Sit quietly and reflect on the skills that have been discussed in this section. How many of them are applicable in your health-care setting? To what degree do you feel that you have had training in those that are applicable?

Now ask yourself the following questions.

- What do I need to do to enhance my therapeutic skills?
- Am I an effective listener?
- If not, what gets in the way of my listening effectively?
- Am I an effective counsellor?
- What degree of structure do I use in counselling?
- If I was asked to facilitate a group tomorrow, what would I have to do now?

PART THREE

Communication and Colleagues: Organizational skills

Introduction

All health-care professionals work in organizations. Many find themselves faced with a managerial function at some point. In Part Three, various organizational skills are explored.

Chapter 7 identifies some of the specific skills that arise in management: managing time and people, delegation and appraisal. In Chapter 8, a range of skills to do with running and organizing meetings is considered. Many people loathe meetings and see them as a waste of time. How can they be used to ensure that everyone benefits? How can they be organized to ensure that nobody's time is wasted? All health professionals need a range of strategies for coping with meetings.

In the final chapter in this section, the question of interviewing is addressed. Again, most health professionals find that they have to organize interviews, often as part of the appointment process. The other side to the issue of interviewing is being interviewed. In Chapter 9 the process of being a candidate at an interview is also addressed and the chapter closes with details of how to write and maintain a CV.

Management skills   7

AIMS OF THE CHAPTER

The following issues and skills are discussed.

- Managing time
- Managing people
- Delegation

Part of being a health professional is managing people and time. This chapter explores some aspects of management with particular emphasis on structuring time and managing work.

MANAGING TIME

The first aspect of managing your time is observing how you use it. The best way to do this is to keep a log or journal which identifies what you do and how long it takes you. The following is an example of one page of a log that I kept. Note how *everything* is logged. Note, too, the interruptions and the inefficiencies. Simply keeping a log of this sort can help you to organize your time better. If you can, keep such a log for at least a week and preferably two.

9.03	Sit down at desk and review three papers. Decide not to do anything about them at present.
9.15	Turn on computer. While it is booting up, make phone call.
9.22	Review and answer some e-mail.
9.26	Phone call answered and query dealt with.
9.28	Return to answering e-mail.
9.35	Secretary brings in opened mail. Decide to abandon e-mail for present. Review pile of mail.
9.46	Visit machine in corridor for soft drink.

9.47	Take phone call, promise to look up information and phone back.
9.50	Divide mail into 'immediate' and 'later' piles.
9.55	Begin to dictate replies to letters.
10.01	Phone call answered and query dealt with.
10.03	Return to dictation.
10.10	One letter requires details from a file. Look up file and find information.
10.15	Return to dictation.

Notice some of the things that waste time. I could, for instance, have diverted my phone to my secretaries and thus had a 'phone-free' period. Later, I could have made a number of phone calls together. Alternatively, I could have used my answerphone to collect messages during the first part of the morning. Notice, too, the tendency for some things to be started and not finished. I began to answer my e-mail but did not continue. Also, I worked through my post twice – first, I 'reviewed' it and then I separated it into two piles. While the 'piles' idea is a good one, this can be done straight away. Notice that no really productive work was undertaken for nearly an hour!

The next stage is to identify your main objectives. The log should help you to see what tasks you carry out most frequently. The point is to identify what you need to do most urgently. Look through your log and try to identify what sorts of tasks you do in a week. Then, set down the three most important tasks for next week. Now, fill in a timetable for the week, mapping in, first, those three important tasks. An example of an outline timetable might be as follows:

Time	Monday	Tuesday	Wednesday	Thursday	Friday
9.00–10.00					
10.00–11.00					
11.00–12.00					
12.00–13.00	lunch	lunch	lunch	lunch	lunch
13.00–14.00					
14.00–15.00					
15.00–16.00					
16.00–17.00					

There are certain features to bear in mind when drawing up a timetable of this sort. First, account for each hour of your time at work. If you do not, you will not get an accurate picture of your use of time. Second, be realistic about your time allocation to the tasks you have planned but do not be overgenerous to yourself.

Having filled in the important tasks for the week, begin to sketch in the others. An important point here is to only programme about 60% of your time. Allow yourself 'travelling time' between tasks. Also allow yourself some free time. If you 'book' free time in this way, you are more likely to take it. If you do not, you will find things to fit the time that you have at your disposal. Also, when you work with the timetable, stick to the timings as far as possible. If you find that an appointment runs short of the time you have allowed, make a note of the fact and give yourself some extra free time. Do not bring forward an appointment unless absolutely necessary. If you do, you will not be able to monitor your use of time so accurately. Work with your new timetable for another week.

During the time that you use the timetable, you will begin to see patterns forming. Where did you underestimate? Where did you allow too much time? How long did you spend doing unexpected paperwork? Had you allowed for things like opening mail and writing reports? Also, was your day punctuated with making phone calls? If so, consider programming some time into each day which you allocate as 'telephone time'. Then, try to do all your phoning in that time. This sounds a simple solution to a difficult problem but it is surprising how much time can be saved by dealing with most of your calls in one period.

If you take a lot of incoming calls, consider using an answerphone. During busy periods, have the answerphone on at all times and answer the calls that are left in a batch (during your telephone time). Clearly, whether or not you can do this will depend on the sort of work you can do. If you deal with numerous non-urgent calls, this may save you valuable time.

If you find that you are grossly under- or overestimating time allocation to a particular task, log the time taken for that task alone. The following grid can help here.

Date				
Time	Estimated Time	Actual Time	Activity	Why?

With this grid, you note down the time that the task starts and the time that you estimate it will take. On completion of the task, you jot down the actual time that was taken. In the final column, you write the reason for the under- or overestimation. In this way, you carefully monitor your work and your use of time. Once you have mastered your estimation of time more accurately, you can return to your timetable.

The other way of monitoring your time is to keep a To Do list. These are widely available as pre-printed pads but the following example shows you how to draw one up on scrap paper.

TO DO LIST	
Order	Task
2.	See Mrs H.
4.	Drop suit at cleaners.
3.	Attend support group if possible.
1.	Write report for P.K.

The important thing with the To Do list is to get used to using it quickly and to keep using it. Do not allow it to become a time-wasting exercise itself. I once worked with a colleague who seemed to spend the day drawing up new and revised To Do lists, to the exclusion of other work.

Godefroy and Clark (1989) suggest the following points for ensuring that you manage your time effectively.

- Programme no more than ten items per day.
- Divide complex and demanding tasks into more easily programmable sub-activities.
- Learn to make an accurate estimate of the time needed for each task.
- Be ambitious, but don't overload yourself.
- Programme only 60% of your time.
- Revise your plan regularly.
- Finish each task before going on to the next.

Their last item is important. It is easy to get caught up in what has been called the 'busy syndrome' (Bond, 1986) in which you are so swamped by things to do that you only half do a number of tasks. This causes you further anxiety and further work and leads, in turn, to greater inefficiency. Sometimes it is just a question of taking a deep breath and making a start on the pile!

Before you go any further, look through the following list of factors that may stop you organizing your time effectively and identify the ones that particularly apply to you.

- I don't identify priorities.
- I don't have long- and short-term goals.
- I tend to say 'Yes' to everyone.
- I don't organize my day.
- I keep two diaries.
- I don't keep a diary at all.
- I lack motivation.

- I feel stressed.
- I am burnt out.
- I spend too much time on the phone.
- I spend too much time with particular clients/patients.
- I avoid the things I don't like doing.
- I take very long breaks.
- I usually arrive late.
- I take a long time to 'come round' in the morning.
- I often do useless tasks.
- I take on other people's work.
- I rewrite reports very frequently.
- I write long letters.
- I always have someone else check my work.
- I like to discuss what I do before I do it.
- I don't have the equipment I need to do the job.
- I like meeting other people, socially, during work time.
- I can't concentrate for long periods.

Once you have read through this list, add some of your own factors to it. Then act on the extended list.

MANAGING PEOPLE

The key to successful management in the health services is the management of people. There are many books about people management available in the shops. In this section, the main aim is to get you to think about the way in which you interrelate with work colleagues in your particular health-care setting. Good social skills and the ability to listen to other people seem crucial here, as does the need to be appropriately assertive. As a means of thinking about your own skills in managing people, consider the following questions.

- How do you greet your colleagues?
- How do you address them?
- How approachable are you?
- Do colleagues come to you with their personal as well as work-related problems?
- What do you imagine other people think of your work?
- Are you able to ask them?
- Do they see you as 'the boss' or as a 'colleague'?
- Do you consciously cultivate a management style?
- What do you do when you are angry with other people?
- How do you handle other people's distress?
- How do you manage the breaking of bad news?
- Do you think carefully before you discuss things with your colleagues?

- How much of what other people do is negotiable with them?
- Do you believe in letting other people do what they want?
- Do you think that you should 'manage' other people?
- Would you say that your style was 'directive' or 'person centred'?
- How did you learn the style that you use?
- How could you be more effective with other people?
- Do you know your weak spots?
- Would you say that you are defensive?
- Do you encourage other people?
- Do others take part in most decisions that are made?

Considering these questions can help you to decide what changes (if any) you need to make to your style of helping and managing others. You may also want to think about your own training and development. In a management position it is easy to be so caught up with the management process and with encouraging other people that your own needs and wants get overlooked. Think about two aspects to such training: formal educational courses (such as diploma courses and courses such as the Master of Business Administration) and one-off short courses or study days. The former can help in the long term to make you more effective in your work. The latter can be great morale boosters and motivators.

MANAGING YOURSELF

Management is never particularly easy. The stress of taking responsibility, looking after others and trying to meet the goals of the organization takes its toll. It is vital that you also look after yourself, as well as looking after others. Dorothy Rowe, a psychologist with a special interest in depression, offers the following 'ten short cuts to happiness'. These are not particularly 'simple' short cuts and may take some working at. However, they are also likely to work.

1. Treat yourself as your own best friend.
2. If disliking yourself is a tough habit to break, practise acting *as if* you are your own best friend. One morning you'll wake up and find that you are.
3. Write a description of yourself as your best friend would write it.
4. Make a list of all the pleasurable things you can do just for you alone and do at least one every day.
5. Every day do something physical (a short, brisk walk is enough), something intellectual (like reading a newspaper article right through) and something spiritual (like listening to music, reading a poem, watching the trees and the sky).
6. Limit how much time you spend thinking about the past and the future and concentrate on enjoying the present. (If you find this hard to do take up yoga and learn how.)
7. Write an account of you and your 'story'.

8. Identify the immutable assumptions your story is based on, like 'If I don't win, I'm no good'.
9. Create some alternative assumptions, especially ones which give you more choices, e.g. change repeated thoughts like 'People like me can't/don't do that' to 'Try anything once'.
10. Now see how many alternative stories you can construct and decide which one you'd like to live.

(Rowe, 1996).

Rowe suggests that we can write the recipe for happiness as follows.

- Accept and value yourself.
- Accept that we live in a world where things happen by chance.

Perhaps one of the marks of maturity as a person is living with ambiguity and appreciating that we do not live in a 'just world'. We have to learn to tolerate the fact that things go wrong, that we do not always get from life what we would like and that we are not always able to 'get things right'.

DELEGATION

Most managers, unless they work in a very small team and are part of a well-defined organization and structure, need to delegate. Many managers, however, are not particularly good at delegation. As a simple rule of thumb, the following questions can help to identify the areas of work that can be delegated. Try to answer them now.

- What do you *have* to do?
- What do others *have* to do?
- What are you doing at present that others *could* do?
- What are you doing at present that others might *do better*?

Through writing notes about the nature of your work and the work of others that you supervise, it becomes clearer how to allocate work fairly to other people. Clearly, it is important that you do not delegate all your work to others. Nor should you dodge unpleasant tasks that *should* be carried out by you. Also, it is essential that your staff do not get overloaded with work and that work is fairly and reasonably allocated. At this point you might want to reflect on the degree to which you appreciate the work load of those with whom you work – at this moment. Do you have difficulty in recalling who does what? Are you unclear about how many tasks other colleagues are engaged in? Part of the process of successful delegation is making sure that you are asking the right person to carry out the task. The subset of that issue is the degree to which you understand and appreciate the nature of the job that that person is doing at present. Here are some reasons for *not* delegating.

- *I want the thanks for a particular task.* This is a fairly egotistical reason for not delegating and one associated more frequently with a younger or newer manager. Part of the process of managing is to encourage others to develop both personally and within the organization.
- *I know what needs to be done.* Others will, too, if you allow them the chance.
- *I don't want mistakes made.* Again, people who are trusted to work and find out solutions to problems are more likely to be better decision makers in the future. An organization which encourages some 'mistake making' is likely to be a healthy one. Most people learn, to some degree, from their mistakes.
- *People may not want to do the things that I delegate to them.* But this is why you are a manager. Your task is to 'sell' ideas to others and also to be assertive enough to ask them to do those things that they may not want to.
- *I want to be popular.* You will be more popular if you are seen to be assertive, fair and consistent. You will not be particularly popular if you are seen as the person who takes on everything yourself and delegates nothing.

The following issues are important once you have decided to delegate.

- Be clear about *what* you are delegating. Is it a task or is it also the responsibility that goes with that task?
- Set a time limit. People work better when they are clear about how much time they have to complete a task. Be realistic about the amount of time you allocate.
- Be sure the other person knows what has been delegated. Be sure, too, that they know whether or not responsibility for the task has also been delegated.
- Be available if help is required but do not constantly check on progress.

Eyre (1993) offers a useful summary of how delegation should be planned and implemented. He suggests that a delegator must:

- determine what tasks are most suitable for delegation, both from the point of view of their own overall work responsibilities and from the point of view of the organizational benefit;
- select very carefully the subordinate to whom authority is to be delegated, from the aspect of the delegate's competence and their personal qualities;
- specify very carefully the duties to be taken over and the limits of the authority invested in the delegate;
- ensure that the delegate is properly acquainted with the above and provide guidance and training if and when necessary;
- ensure that the authority delegated is fully commensurate with the responsibilities the delegate has to assume. It is not only useless but also patently unjust to require duties to be properly performed without at the same time giving sufficient authority to accomplish them;
- allow the delegate to carry out their duties with as little interference as possible, having ascertained that they are competent to perform them. After all, the purpose of delegation is to free the delegator for other things. Further, the

responsibility underaken should increase the competence, self-confidence and potential of the delegate.
- despite the above, ensure that some form of checking is instituted to ascertain that the delegate is performing effectively. As has been pointed out, delegation does not absolve the delegator from responsibility for the work delegated. It has been said, with truth, that inspection is the corollary of delegation.

SUMMARY

Managing time and managing people are two key elements in the communication system of any organization. This is as true in the health professions as it is in business. This chapter has explored practical ways to enhance your time and people skills.

References

Bond, M. (1986) *Stress and Self-Awareness*, Heinemann, London.
Eyre, E.C. (1993) *Mastering Basic Management*, Macmillan, London.
Godefroy, C.H. and Clark, J. (1989) *The Complete Time Management System*, Gower, London.
Rowe, D. (1996) The escape from depression. The Sunday Review, *Independent on Sunday*, 31st March.

8

Meeting skills

AIMS OF THE CHAPTER

The following skills and issues are discussed.

- Identifying types of meetings
- Planning the meeting
- The agenda
- Running the meeting
- Coping with contingencies
- Notes and minutes

Health professionals are required to attend and run numerous meetings. Why do you go to meetings? What sorts of meetings do you go to? What are their functions? Before anything else happens, it is essential to know what *sort* of meeting you are being asked to organize and run.

Williams (1984) identifies six main sorts of meetings.

1. *Command meeting.* This is the meeting called by a manager to pass on information or to exercise control over staff. This sort of meeting may be common in the health professions.
2. *Selling meeting.* In this sort of meeting, an individual or group of people are engaged in trying to convince others of the need for or the validity of a planned project.
3. *Advisory meeting.* This meeting is called to exchange ideas or information or to seek opinions.
4. *Negotiating meeting.* Here, the object is to reach a compromise or agreement over a matter in dispute. This type of meeting may be called when there are changes happening in an organization or where job roles are changing.
5. *Problem-solving meeting.* This is called to tackle a specific problem or series of problems that face a group of health professionals or an organization.
6. *Support meeting.* Here, people meet to help each other, offer support and often, express feelings and emotions. Such meetings are often organized by or for relatives or those suffering in particular life situations.

Whilst this may not be an exhaustive classification of all possible types of meetings, it is clear that the aims of a particular meeting will depend upon that meeting's purpose. As a variety of issues regarding group facilitation and therapy have already been addressed, the types of meeting methods discussed here deal with more formal meetings. Thus, the sorts of meetings that will require the skills described in this chapter are more likely to be the command, negotiating and problem-solving ones.

PLANNING THE MEETING

Having decided what sort of meeting you want to call, there are other considerations to make. A shortlist of these would be:

- Who needs to be at the meeting? This is not always as easy to answer as it might seem. It is tempting to invite the whole department to every meeting. Think about this carefully and only invite the essential people.
- Where will the meeting be held? Is the room that you have in mind large enough or even too large? Do you have to book ahead to make sure that the room is available?
- What is the purpose of the meeting? Your meeting might be called for any of the following purposes.
    – Information giving
    – Obtaining information
    – Creating and sharing ideas
    – Departmental decision making
    – Patient/client policy making
    – Presenting proposals
    – Questioning other people's proposals
    – Discussing patient/client progress.
- How will you inform people of the meeting? A frequent cry amongst health professionals is that they did not know that a meeting was to be held.
- Who will chair the meeting? Godefroy and Clark (1989) suggest the following method of selecting a chairman if the issue has not been resolved prior to the meeting. Once the meeting is in session, you count up to three. At three, each participant points to another. The person with the most votes is elected to the chair. The rest of this chapter, however, anticipates that *you* will be the chairman.

AGENDA

It is very frustrating to arrive at a meeting to find that no agenda has been set. Set it well in advance of the meeting. If necessary, phone or circulate a list to colleagues for agenda items. Then draw up a list of priorities. It may help if you think in terms of:

- what *must* be on the agenda;
- what *should* be on the agenda;
- what *could* be on the agenda.

The *must* items will naturally go straight on the final agenda. After that, it is a question of allocating time to each item and deciding what else can go on it. The point of this sort of planning is that it can help you focus very clearly on how much time you spend on items in the meeting itself. A little forethought can pay great dividends in the meeting proper.

THE ROLE OF THE CHAIRMAN

There is no formal mechanism for choosing a chairman of a meeting. Most chairmen, though, are voted into the position by the committee or the meeting. Developing the work of Eyre (1993), it is possible to identify the following duties of the meeting chairman.

The chairman should:

1. be satisfied that he has been appropriately elected to the position and holds it rightfully;
2. ensure that the meeting is properly convened, appropriately constituted and that the people at the meeting have a right to be there;
3. make sure that a quorum is present. Usually, the number that makes up a quorum will be made clear in standing orders or identified in a document about the consitution of the committee;
4. make sure that the minutes of the previous meeting have been prepared, circulated to committee members, read by them and worked through by all committee members at the start of the meeting. Once this has been done, the minutes can be signed as a true record of the previous meeting;
5. see that items are worked through in the order of the agenda;
6. give everyone an opportunity to contribute to the meeting as they see fit. The chairman should, in particular, make sure that less vocal members of the committee have their say;
7. in the case of dispute, act quickly and decisively;
8. reject issues that are not on the agenda. Although there is usually an agenda item known as 'any other business', this should not be taken as an opportunity to introduce issues quite outside the remit of the committee;
9. insist that all communication is directed 'through the chair'. Committee members should not, generally, address each other directly. Instead, their points should be addressed to the other person via the chairman. It is sometimes necessary for the chairman to remind committee members of this rule;

10. put motions and amendments to the vote and make sure that the appropriate voting procedure is adhered to;

11. in the event of a tied vote, use the casting vote. Normally, the chairman votes to maintain the status quo;

12. if there is no particular voting procedure, identify the 'sense of the meeting' and make it clear to the secretary what has been agreed on any given issue. This 'sense' can be checked with the committee members as necessary;

13. set a date for the next meeting. In practice, it is better to set *all* the dates for meetings well in advance. If a 'next meeting' date is set at the close of a particular meeting, any member who is not able to attend on that occasion may find that they are also unable to attend on the date fixed for the next. In this way, it is quite possible to miss a string of meetings simply as a result of missing one.

14. declare the meeting closed;

15. make sure that adequate notes of the meeting are kept by the secretary and check these before they are circulated to members.

RUNNING THE MEETING

Think carefully about how you will run your meeting. First, start exactly on time and do not be too friendly and accepting towards latecomers. This tends to reinforce two things: it makes it appear that timing is not particularly important to you and it gives the appearance of sloppiness. If you cannot be seen to be working to time at the beginning of the meeting, can you be trusted to work through the agenda and finish on time?

Work through your prepared agenda, keeping fairly rigidly to the time scale that you worked out when you wrote it. If you feel that you are unlikely to get through the whole agenda, negotiate changes as the need arises. This is not, however, a particularly good policy. If you can, stick to the agenda.

Pay close attention to what each person has to say, whilst keeping up a 'wide sweep' of attention to the other members of the meeting. Make sure that everyone gets a hearing and that they are satisfied with the responses that they invoke. Be prepared to sum up some of the longer comments and check with the person who has spoken to make sure that your summary is accurate. Be wary, however, of allowing the person a 'second breath', during which they repeat what they have said before.

Bring things to a clear conclusion and make sure that at the end of each item, the *action* element of a decision is noted. Make sure that everyone is clear about their responsibilities after the meeting. Whilst all decisions will be minuted, those minutes will not be read until later. People need to leave a meeting knowing what is expected of them.

COPING WITH CONTINGENCIES

Not all meetings run to plan. A variety of ploys can be used by people at meetings, either consciously or otherwise, to disrupt the proceedings. The following issues have been identified as common 'disrupters'.

- *Late arrival*. Here, the member of the meeting arrives late and takes some time to settle. There is usually considerable shuffling of papers and moving of seats as the person sits down. One way to counteract this behaviour is to insist on people arriving on time. Another is to ask the late arriver to take their place quickly so as to minimally disrupt the meeting. If the behaviour persists from meeting to meeting, the chairman may have to talk to the late arriver in private.
- *Pairing.* Here, two members of the meeting quietly collude with each other. Sometimes they speak almost subvocally to each other and make 'asides' about other members of the meeting. Another behaviour associated with pairing is note passing between two people sitting together. It is usually a sign of regression and can be a direct threat to the chair. Sometimes, though, it is a sign of boredom and the chairman who encounters a lot of pairing should reconsider the length or number of meetings that are held.
- *Walking out*. One fairly legitimate reason for a member to walk out is that they have a prior engagement elsewhere. Consider, though, why this is happening. Has the meeting run on too long? Did it start late and is it now running late? If so, remedial action needs to be taken in the future. Alternatively, the person may plan to leave early, thus attracting the meeting's attention. As with other such manoeuvres, the chairman may have to talk to this person away from the meeting. More difficult to handle is the person who walks out of the meeting in an emotionally charged state. This must be dealt with in context. Sometimes, it is appropriate to ask someone to follow them and talk to them. At other times, it is better to merely allow the person to leave. It is rarely a good idea to abandon the meeting, although a short 'cooling off' break may be appropriate.
- *Delaying*. Here, one or more members take time over small issues that everyone else feels could be dealt with more rapidly. It is important to discriminate between delaying and appropriate attention to detail. It should not be assumed that all detailed questioning and discussion is a symptom of delaying.
- *The straw person syndrome*. This is a special case of delaying. Here, a detailed 'case' is built up by one or more of the meeting members, a case that has little evidence or relevance. An example of how such straw person arguments start is as follows.

'Supposing if some of our case workers are taken out of the department and then we are all rehoused. Supposing, then, that the government changes its policy on hospital admissions and then we find ourselves short of staff ...'

The point about the straw person argument is that it uses so many 'ifs' that the picture painted is almost completely unrelated to likelihood or reality. Sometimes, in the debate that follows, the straw person debater uses the 'Yes but ...' ploy (Berne, 1974). To every objection to their argument, they say something like 'Yes, but what happens if ...?'. One way of coping with such a scenario is to gently unpack the person's argument with logic and invitations to address the *likelihood* of the scenario. The straw person syndrome is not always easy to deal with and is yet another variety of delaying tactics.

- *Overtalking*. Some people like to make themselves heard at meetings. Others like to take over the meeting. The 'overtalker' must be differentiated from the person who has a particular interest in the topic on the agenda. The overtalker usually has to say more than anyone else on *every* topic. Such a person needs firm direction from the chair and the chairman may want to direct the order of speaking, thus: 'Sarah first, then Peter ...'.

NOTES AND MINUTES

It is important to establish early on in the proceedings who will take the minutes of the meeting. Whilst some chairpersons like this to be a voluntary task, it is important that the chairperson does not find themselves doing the job, whilst trying to chair the meeting. It may be preferable, if possible, to take on secretarial help. It is vital that whoever takes the minutes has either had experience of doing it or has a clear idea of how to lay them out once they are taken.

A final issue is how or whether to take personal notes during a meeting. If the meeting is properly minuted, detailed notes should not be necessary. However, it is important that everyone brings their diaries to meetings in order to set the times and dates of future meetings. It is usually better to set such times and dates for at least the next three meetings. Also, members who have certain tasks to do before the publication of the minutes may want to jot down the elements involved in those tasks.

Two methods of note taking can be recommended. First is the style which makes use of separate 'blocks' of words, illustrated below. The advantage of this method is that it makes it immediately clear where one note finishes and the next one starts. It is also a very easy method to get used to and many people use it for note taking in educational settings.

Note-taking Style 1

1. Starting tomorrow, all staff will have to draw up personal plans for coping with emergencies. These should include the following:

- date and time
- name(s)
- nature of the emergency
- who reported to
- other action taken.

Remember to work on this tonight and draft out plan.

2. Peter is to take on the role of team leader in the psychiatric division. All psychiatric referrals should be made through him in the future. How will this affect Sarah and David? Discuss this with them pronto!

3. New Green Paper to be distributed through the department. Advised to read the sections on changes in child care. It may be worth getting a copy of this. Ring bookshop tomorrow or consider library copy. Will the students need a session on this?

The second style of note taking is the well-known 'spider's web' method. Here, a central theme is jotted down in the middle of the notepad. Then, 'spokes' are developed out of the central theme and 'branches' added to the spokes. The advantage of this method is that it allows you to write as you think. It also allows you to take in a wide range of details in one go. The disadvantage is that it often looks untidy and this may upset tidier people. An example of this style is illustrated below. The style is also widely used in education and learning settings.

Finally, it is important to file such notes. It is worth considering keeping a 'meetings file' in the form of a ring binder divided into sections for each of the

Note-taking Style 2

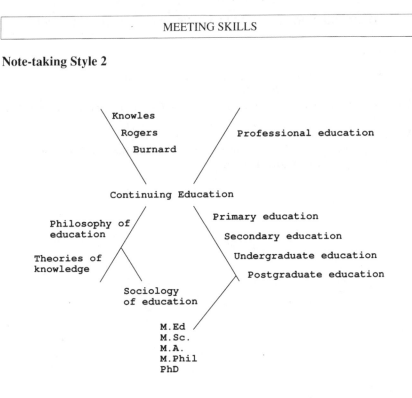

meetings that you go to or chair. Even more organized is to have one file for meetings that you chair and another for those where you are a member. If you keep such files, you can take them with you to each meeting and make reference to previous agendas and prior note taking. This tends to be a much better approach than merely dropping all your notes and agendas into a file in a filing cabinet. As we have noted throughout this chapter, the key element in effective meeting management is *structure*. Structure in note taking and filing will also pay off in making better use of your time and resources.

SUMMARY

This chapter has discussed skills related to running a variety of meetings but particularly the more formal, chaired meeting. By its nature, the chaired meeting is highly structured. You are advised to use that structure to make your meetings productive. The structure can also give you confidence when the going gets rough.

References

Berne, E. (1974) *Games People Play*, Penguin, Harmondsworth.

Eyre, E.C. (1993) *Mastering Basic Management*, Macmillan, London.

Godefroy, C.H. and Clark, J. (1989) *The Complete Time Management System*, Gower, London.

Williams, G.L. (1984) Observing and recording meetings, in *Conducting Small-Scale Investigations in Educational Management*, (eds J. Bell, T. Bush, A. Fox, J. Goodey and S. Goulding), Harper & Row, London.

9

Interview skills

AIMS OF THE CHAPTER

The following skills and issues are discussed.
- Selection
- Conducting the interview
- Decision making
- Being interviewed
- Preparing a CV

SELECTION

The first stage in setting up the process of selection interviews is the placing of advertisements. First define your post, then write the advert. What you must be clear about is what the job entails and what sort of people you want applying for it. Once you have done that, it is important to make sure that all the information that a prospective employee will want is in the advert. Issues here include:

- the job title;
- a short summary of what the job involves;
- the salary scale;
- who may apply;
- to whom they might apply (along with an address and phone number).

Whilst it is easy to be overinclusive in advertisements, it is also possible to be too frugal. Consider, too, the 'tone' of the advertisement. Try to avoid overly formal language. An example of a stilted and formal tone might be:

> Suitably qualified applicants are invited to apply for
> the post of:
> Senior Nurse
>
> Applicants with a recent history of successful management in acute settings will be considered for the above post. The following are essential for this post.
>
> - Registration on the General Part of the Register.
> - A minimum of three years experience in a post of charge nurse or above.
> - Willingness to study for a degree or higher degree.
>
> Suitable applicants may apply, in the first instance, to Mr P. Davies, Director of Personnel, Brigemont Hospital Trust, Brigemont, Somerset. Phone 01657–3434 ext. 231.

Consider ways in which such an advert could be made more appealing. First of all, try to avoid ambiguous and superfluous phrases such as 'suitably qualified applicants' (are unsuitably qualified ones likely to apply?) and 'with a recent history of' (this sounds as though the applicants might be expected to have a *medical* history) and 'in the first instance' (what exactly does this mean?). Also, consider offering your candidates the full name of the person that they can contact (Peter Davies) and recommend that they can contact him for an informal visit. Generally try to be welcoming in your approach to advertisement writing. Remember that your advertisement helps to form the first impression that people have of your organization. People other than job applicants read adverts too.

SHORTLISTING

It is usual for shortlisting to be carried out by a panel of people. It is often best for this process to be chaired and run along fairly structured lines. First, the shortlisting group draws up a list of criteria for the job. Once this is agreed upon, it is a relatively simple clerical task to work through the applications and screen out those that do not meet those criteria. In the second round, detailed discussion and reading of application forms can take place to determine the final shortlist. It is useful if each person draws up a list of three people that they would like to see interviewed and then, in turn, each person justifies the three that they have chosen. From this process, the final list is devised.

Another consideration is the question of whether or not references are taken up prior to interviewing. Once that decision has been made, the next is to determine whether or not those references will be read by the interviewing panel before the interviews. Some panels prefer to interview first and read the references after they have settled on one or two possible candidates for the job.

THE INTERVIEW

Some people loathe the prospect of interviewing almost as much as they do the process of being interviewed. A little careful planning can help here. Considerations that need to be made prior to the interview are these.

- Where will the interviewees gather and who will meet them to settle them there?
- Who will call the interviewee and will that person then introduce them to each member of the panel?
- How will the interview proceed? A traditional approach is for each of the interviewers to ask two or three questions of each person (usually the same questions). This method of interview does not allow for any real interaction between interviewer and interviewee. A more imaginative approach is to allocate a certain amount of time to each interviewer and to allow them to develop a rapport and discussion with the interviewee.
- Who will invite the interviewee to ask questions at the end of the interview and who will round off the process and thank the candidate for coming?
- What will be the standard response to the question of when the outcome of the interview will be made known to interviewees?

If these issues can be decided upon through discussion, prior to the interview, the whole process can be more successful. Also, if the interview panel is large, it is important that it is chaired. The chairperson might be a contributing interviewer or may limit their interaction to the chairing process.

It is helpful if the interview also follows a reasonably formal structure, even if the discussion during the interview is fairly unstructured. Typically, the following points are covered during a job interview.

- The applicant's account of their education and work prior to the application.
- Reasons for wanting the job.
- Strengths and weaknesses.
- Special factors that the applicant can bring to the post.
- Financial and logistic issues (when the applicant would be able to start work, entry on the salary scale and so forth).

Eyre (1993) identifies the following 'five-point plan' that is often used in selection interviews.

1. *Physical requirements*. These include age, height, eyesight, dexterity, etc.
2. *Intelligence*. This includes issues such as the ability to think clearly and critically.
3. *Aptitudes*. This is concerned with the candidate's appropriateness for the job and any qualities that they may have that will ensure an appropriate fitness for purpose.
4. *Attainments*. These cover the candidate's educational and training achievements.

5. *Personality and temperament.* These refer to the candidate's appropriateness for the job in terms of outlook, ability to work with others and other 'personal' qualities.

Ideally, the interview should be a two-way process. Not only does the interview panel interview the applicant but the applicant also has the chance to discuss the job and their suitability for it. The more formal the interview, the less likelihood there is of a productive discussion occurring. If only highly structured questions are asked, only 'best performance' answers will be offered. Remember that the candidate will have rehearsed most of the standard interview questions. The more informal, open-ended interviews (within a more formal outer structure) are more likely to yield in-depth answers and insights.

Most people who have conducted interviews are familiar with the idea of starting with a few simple questions to get the candidate talking. These usually relate to travelling to the interview or to the candidate's familiarity with the area. It is useful to notice the candidate's body language or non-verbal aspects of communication and to time the 'deeper' and more penetrating questions with visible signs of relaxation. Indicators here may be:

- uncrossing of previously crossed arms and legs;
- increased levels of eye contact;
- smiling;
- increased use of hand gestures;
- change in depth of breathing;
- change of tone in voice.

During the 'body' of the interview, it is helpful if all questions are clear, unambiguous and contain only one question. It is easy, for example, to find yourself asking multiple questions like this: 'How do you cope with stress? Do you find that you can relax fairly easily after work? Or are you a person who tends to take their work home with them? What are your views on this?'. Four questions in one. Instead, make sure that you are clear about what you want to ask. Follow up an initial question with a series of 'open' questions, if necessary, to encourage further discussion. Examples of open questions include:

- What did you do then …?
- How do you feel about that …?
- Can you think of other examples …?
- What do you think of that …?
- How do you do that …?

Open questions should be asked in a supportive and caring manner and not in an inquisitorial way. The aim is for you and the interviewee to get to know each other better. Remember that the person you are interviewing also has to make a decision about whether or not they want to work with you and your colleagues. Again, as an interviewer, you are saying a lot about the organization in which you work.

When the interviewee is answering your questions, make sure that you listen. It is easy, when you are anxious, to get caught up with your own questions to the point that you no longer listen to the answers. An aid to the listening process is suggested by Egan (1990) who offers the following pointers to effective listening behaviour (these are discussed in greater detail in Chapter 4).

- Sit squarely: face the interviewee rather than sitting next to them.
- Sit in an 'open' position and try not to fold your arms and legs as this suggests defensiveness.
- Lean slightly towards the other person.
- Maintain reasonable eye contact.
- Relax and resist the temptation to rehearse future questions while you are listening to the interviewee's answers.

DECISION MAKING

Once you have interviewed all the candidates, the decision has to be made as to who you appoint. The option usually exists to decide whether or not you *do* appoint. The factors that will help you in this process are:

- notes that you have taken after each interview. It is not a good plan to make notes during the interview, at least not if you are asking the questions. It is sometimes reasonable for those not asking the questions to take notes;
- discussion evolving out of a 'round' conducted at the end of the interviews. In this activity, each interviewer in turn says who they felt to be the best two candidates and why. No further discussion occurs until each person has spoken;
- re-reading (or reading for the first time, as appropriate) of the references.

It is usually a good idea to submit all decisions to a 'devil's advocate' process in which likely candidates are explored through the question of 'why they should *not* be appointed' as well as through the more usual one of 'why they *should* be appointed'. This allows for clarity of decision making and the covering of most of the issues governing appointment.

BEING INTERVIEWED

The other side of the interview process is that of being interviewed. As noted above, it is by no means clear which aspect of the process provokes the most anxiety. Some people find the business of conducting interviews very traumatic. This knowledge can help you to overcome your own preinterview nerves.

Presenting yourself

There are certain fairly simple things that you can do to ensure that you are seen in your best light. These include the following.

- Make sure that the interviewers have what they asked for. Ensure that your application form or introductory letter is complete. If you are asked to present a CV, make sure that it is properly filled out. How to prepare a CV and what to put in it is covered below.
- Do your homework. Know something about the organization in which you are being interviewed. If possible, always make an informal (although scheduled) visit prior to the interview but not on the same day as the interview.
- Practise the interview process with a colleague or friend. Ask them to field you a number of difficult questions and anticipate your answers. Practise answering questions with concise but accurate replies. On the one hand, no interviewer wants you to be monosyllabic but on the other, interviewers tend not to like having to interrupt you so that they can get on with the next question.
- Look your best. It is usually best to dress reasonably formally (but not flashily) for interviews. It is a mistake to think that people do not notice clothes, that they should accept you for what you are or that they no longer take clothes and appearance into consideration. Spend some time thinking about how you will look but do not spend so much time on it that you fail to relax during the interview. Do not try to stun the interview panel.
- Arrive in plenty of time. You can always stop for coffee near to the interview site. If it is inevitable that you will be late, however, phone through to inform the interview panel.
- Prepare some short questions that you can ask when approached by the panel. Do not ask 'impossible' questions ('Could you tell me the history of this unit?'). Keep your questions simple and make sure that they can be answered by the interviewer in a couple of sentences. If you have real anxieties about the job, make sure that these are discussed during your questioning period. Remember that the interview should be a two-way process: you should be finding out about the people who are interviewing you.

Finally, make sure that you really want the job for which you are applying. Perhaps you cannot always make up your mind before you go for interview but it is a mistake to use interviews merely as 'experience' and to go through an interview process with no intention of taking the job if you are offered it. Remember that many interviewers will ask you if you *will* take the job if it is offered you.

PREPARING A CV

The CV or curriculum vitae is just that: a 'life curriculum' or description of your life to date. Think carefully about what you put in it. It is usually a good idea to keep a copy of your CV in your possession at all times and to update it regularly. That way, when you apply for a job, there is no problem in remembering what you have and have not done. If you use a computer and word processor, it is useful to keep your CV as a file and to add to it as new things happen to you. You may want to keep a 'short version' which summarizes the essential parts of your personal history, as well as the full version. The short version can be a useful aid to filling in application forms and may be asked for during applications for jobs, grants or scholarships.

CVs typically cover the following subject areas.

- Name
- Address
- Work address
- Date of birth
- Age
- Marital status
- Place of birth
- Nationality
- Current post
- Secondary, professional and higher education
- Other professional training (short courses, management courses, etc.)
- Professional employment
- Summary of responsibilities in present post
- Committee membership
- Other professional activities (membership of unions, clubs, associations, editorial boards, external examining, etc.)
- Other activities (governorship of schools, membership of other organizations, etc.)
- Miscellaneous section (driving licence, word-processing skills, etc.)
- Research
- Conference papers
- Publications (books, chapters in books, articles in referred journals, articles in other journals).

Not all of these headings will be necessary or appropriate to everyone's CV but you should aim at making yours as comprehensive as possible. Make sure that all the dates are correct and that the spelling and layout are appropriate. At the end of the CV it is sometimes correct to include the names and addresses of two or three people who will write references for you. Make sure that you ask those people's permission to quote their names before you do so.

SUMMARY

This chapter has considered the skills involved in the two sides of interviewing: the process of interviewing other people and the process of being interviewed. It has illustrated how, through simple structure, the business of applying for jobs can be made less anxiety provoking for all concerned. All the skills described here can also be applied in other interview situations: applications for grants, scholarships and fellowships to name but three.

References

Egan, G. (1990) *The Skilled Helper*, 4th edn, Brooks/Cole, Pacific Grove, California.
Eyre, E.C. (1993) *Mastering Basic Management*, Macmillan, London.

Skills check: Part Three

Sit quietly and reflect on the skills that have been discussed in this section. How many of them are applicable in your health-care setting? To what degree do you feel that you have had training in those that are applicable?

Now ask yourself the following questions.

- What am I like as a manager?
- How organized am I?
- How effectively do I use my time?
- If I was asked to chair a meeting tomorrow, what would I have to do now?

PART FOUR

Communication through Teaching:
Educational skills

Introduction

Education and training techniques in the health profession are changing. The model that is being adopted increasingly is one that recognizes students as adults. In Part Four we explore a range of skills that are important in the education of students. First, the question of teaching skills. If an adult model of education and training is to be used, *facilitation* skills rather than traditional 'telling' techniques will have to be developed. Chapter 10 explores facilitation and teaching methods.

More and more health-care professionals are called upon to speak about their work, either 'in house' or at conferences and workshops. Chapter 11 considers the practical skills that go towards making an effective and professional presentation.

Computers and computing play an increasing part in health care. Every health-care professional is likely to come into contact with computers at some stage in their career. At present, we are in an interesting stage of our development, where younger people are likely to know more about the subject than more senior colleagues. Many health-care workers will find that their children know more about computers than they do. Chapter 12 explores practical aspects of computing as they relate to studying and researching. Throughout Part Four, the emphasis is on education: lifelong education. No health-care professional, whatever their discipline, can stop studying. We all have to be continual students. There are certain skills that can help us to study, teach and learn more effectively. Part Four examines and explores those skills.

Teaching skills

10

AIMS OF THE CHAPTER

The following skills are discussed.

- Teaching adults
- Using experiential learning methods
- Planning teaching sessions
- Running teaching sessions
- Evaluating learning

TEACHING ADULTS

Being an effective communicator often involves teaching and learning. Staff training, professional education, patient or client information giving all involve the teaching of adults. In this first section, the principles of adult education are explored, as is the concept of experiential learning or learning by experience. The chapter goes on to consider the planning and execution of facilitation sessions in line with modern educational and therapeutic thought. It closes with the consideration of styles of facilitation. The skills and issues discussed in this chapter are relevant to all health-care facilitators whether they are formally designated as such or find themselves teaching others or helping them to reflect on their personal experience.

LEARNING FROM EXPERIENCE

People have always learned from experience. We are all made up of huge numbers of personal experiences that shape us and make us the people we are. However, the idea of experiential learning as an educational concept is relatively recent. It is far more widely known in the concept of therapy, where the whole subject matter of enterprise is human experience.

Experiential learning was developed out of the work of American pragmatic philosopher John Dewey (1916, 1938). Keeton *et al.* (1976) described experiential learning as including learning through the process of living, work experience, skills developed through hobbies and interests and non-formal educational activities. This approach was reflected in the Further Education Unit project report *Curriculum Opportunity* which suggested that experiential learning referred to the knowledge and skills acquired through life, work experience and study (FEU, 1983). This is particularly pertinent to the work of health professionals, almost all of whom develop skills as they work with clients, patients or colleagues.

Pfeiffer and Goodstein (1982) took a different approach by describing an 'experiential learning cycle' which suggested the process of experiential learning. The five stages in their cycle are:

1. experiencing
2. publishing (sharing reactions)
3. processing (discussion of patterns and dynamics)
4. generalizing
5. applying (planning more effective behaviour).

This cycle not only identified a format for organizing experiential learning but also made reference to the way in which people learn through experience.

Kolb (1984) was more explicit about this learning process in his 'experiential learning model' which included the following stages.

1. Concrete experience
2. Observations
3. Formation of abstract concepts and generalizations
4. Testing implications of and reflections on concepts in new situations.

Malcolm Knowles, the American adult educator (Knowles, 1980), gave a different definition of experiential learning. He described the following activities as 'participatory experiential techniques'.

- Group discussion
- Cases
- Critical incidents
- Simulations
- Role play
- Skills practice exercises
- Field practice exercises
- Field projects
- Action projects
- Laboratory methods
- Consultative supervision (coaching)
- Demonstrations
- Seminars

- Work conferences
- Counselling
- Group therapy
- Community development

This all-inclusive list implies that experiential learning techniques excluded only the lecture method or private, individual study and that it was synonymous with participant and discovery learning.

Writers who devised their definitions of experiential learning from the work of Dewey emphasized a cycle of events starting with concrete experience. Kolb's and Pfeiffer and Goodstein's cycles were anticipated by Dewey.

> Thinking includes all of these steps, the sense of a problem, the observation of conditions, the formation and rational elaboration of a suggested conclusion and the active experimental testing.

> (Dewey, 1916, p. 151)

Kolb's notion of transformation of experience and meaning can also be traced back to Dewey, who wrote that:

> In a certain sense every experience should do something to prepare a person for later experiences of a deeper and more expansive quality. That is the very meaning of growth, continuity, reconstruction of experience.

> (Dewey, 1938, p. 47).

This was the influence on experiential learning from the Dewey perspective. The accent was on the primacy of personal experience and on reflection as the tool for changing knowledge and meaning.

Boud and Pascoe (1978) summed up what they considered to be the most important characteristics of experiential education thus.

1. The involvement of each student in their own learning (learning activities need to engage the full attention of a student).
2. The correspondence of the learning activity to the world outside the classroom or the educational institution (the emphasis being on the quality of the experience, not its location).
3. Learner control over the learning experience (learners themselves need to have control over the experience in which they are engaged so that they can integrate it with their own mode of operation in the world and can experience the results of their own decisions).

Boud and Pascoe's list seems to sum up the Dewey approach to learning through experience and through responsibility in the learning process.

It was Carl Rogers (1972) who offered the clearest definition of what experiential or 'significant' learning might be. He identified these elements of experiential learning.

1. It has the quality of personal involvement.
2. It is self-initiated.
3. It is pervasive.
4. It is evaluated by the learner [rather than by educators].
5. Its essence is meaning.

Whilst the final element ('its essence is meaning') is rather unclear, Rogers advocated 'personalized' learning, which he contrasted with 'cognitive learning' or the learning of facts and figures that are imposed by educators. Experiential learning, for Rogers, was learning that was self-initiated and in which the learner's interest and motivation were high. He went on to identify 'assumptions relevant to experiential learning'.

1. Human beings have a natural potential for learning.
2. Significant learning takes place when the subject matter is perceived by the student as having relevance for their own purposes.
3. Much significant learning is acquired through doing.
4. Learning is facilitated when the student participates responsibly in the learning process.
5. Self-initiated learning involving the whole person of the learner – feelings as well as intellect – is the most pervasive and lasting.
6. Creativity in learning is best facilitated when self-criticism and self-evaluation are primary and evaluation by others is of secondary importance.
7. The most socially useful learning in the modern world is the learning of the process of learning, a continuing openness to experience, an incorporation into oneself of the process of change.

Here, Rogers not only spells out the nature of experiential learning but adds dimensions about how he perceives human beings. Rogers argues that human beings function at their best when they are allowed to learn for themselves, a theme that will be familiar to most health professionals. In the end, you can probably only rarely *tell* people important things: mostly, they have to learn for themselves.

EXPERIENTIAL LEARNING AND YOUR ROLE AS A HEALTH PROFESSIONAL

Given the personal nature of learning as discussed above, consider your own learning. Think about the things that you have learned that have *not* involved a teacher or lecturer. You may discover that we learn most of the important things through reflection on our personal experience. If we learn from teachers, then learning occurs most readily when they relate what they are teaching to our own personal experience. As we shall see, the tendency increasingly is to see teachers as 'facilitators of learning' rather than as 'passers on of knowledge'.

Before we go further, however, reflect on this issue of learning from experience. Consider the following list and think about how you learned each of the items on it.

- Relating to others and caring for them.
- Deciding who you like and who you do not.
- Coping with bad news.
- Enjoying your own company.
- Wanting to help other people.
- Liking or not liking yourself.
- Spiritual beliefs or lack of them.
- Sexual identity.
- Personality.

Each of these issues, it is suggested, has more to do with personal experience than it ever does with formal teaching or learning. One of the most important parts of communicating with others is the sharing and developing of personal experience, a recurrent theme throughout this book.

FACILITATION OR TEACHING?

The accent in education in the health professions is changing, with the educational encounter being student centred rather than teacher centred and appropriately adult centred. In this approach, the aim is not to initiate the group participants into particular ways of knowing, as Peters (1969) would argue, but to encourage them to think about their own experience and to transform their personal knowledge and skills through the processes of reflection, discussion and action. In the student-centred approach to learning, the health professional educator acts as a facilitator of learning rather than as a teacher.

The notion of 'teacher' suggests one who passes on knowledge to others, who instructs and manages learning for others. The notion of 'facilitation' has other connotations and these are developed in this chapter alongside the practical issues that need to be addressed if the health professional is to function as a facilitator.

Elizabeth King (1984) offers the following suggestions about the nature of the facilitator's role.

- They must believe students should make their own decisions and think for themselves.
- They must refrain from assuming an authoritative role and adopt a more facilitative and listening position.
- They must accept diversity of race, sex, values, etc. amongst their students.
- They must be willing to accept all viewpoints unconditionally and not impose their personal values on the students. The ability to entertain alternatives and to negotiate no-lose solutions to problems often leads to group decisions that are more beneficial for both the individual and the group.

In the pages that follow, the term 'facilitator' will be used to denote the health professional who is running a group. That group may be a relatively formal learning group, it may be a therapy group or it may be a relatively informal support group. In principle and in practice, the skills involved in helping others to learn from experience turn out to be very similar.

Certain stages in the facilitation process can be described and the facilitator needs to be aware of the processes that can occur in groups. The stages described here are modified from those of Knowles (1975) in his discussion of facilitating learning groups for adults.

Facilitation of learning has more in common with group therapy than it does with teaching. It is recommended that the person who sets out to become a group facilitator gain experience as a member of a number of different sorts of groups before leading one herself. In this way she will not only learn about group processes experientially but she will also see a number of facilitator styles. As Heron (1977) points out, in the early stages of becoming a facilitator it is often helpful to base your style on a facilitator that you have seen in action. Later, the style becomes modified in the light of your own experience and you develop your own approach.

The facilitation of learning has applications in many aspects of the health professional's life. For instance it can be an important part of learning to be a health professional at all. It can also be used as a means of helping clients or patients to explore their problems. It can also be a method of running support groups and self-help groups. The context, then, is sometimes educational, sometimes therapeutic and sometimes supportive.

STAGES IN THE FACILITATION PROCESS

Setting the learning climate

The first aspect of helping adults to learn or explore themselves is the creation of an atmosphere in which adult learners feel comfortable and thus able to learn. Unlike more formal classroom learning, the student-centred approach asks learners to try things out, take some risks and experiment. If this is to happen at all, it needs to be undertaken in an atmosphere of mutual trust and understanding.

The first aspect of the setting of a learning climate is to ensure that the environment is appropriate. Rows of desks and chairs are reminiscent of earlier schooldays. For the adult learning group it is often better and certainly more egalitarian if learners and facilitator sit together in a closed circle of chairs.

In the early stages of a learning group it is useful if the group members spend time getting to know each other. 'Icebreakers' are sometimes used for this purpose. An icebreaker is a simple group activity designed to relax people and allow them to 'let their hair down' a little, thus creating a more relaxed atmosphere, arguably more conducive to learning. An example of an icebreaker is as follows.

The group stands up and group members mill around the room at will. At a signal from the facilitator, each person stops and introduces herself to the nearest person and shares some personal details. Then each person moves on and at a further signal, stops and greets another person in a similar way. This can continue until each group member has met every other, including the facilitator.

Other examples of icebreaking activities can be found elsewhere (Heron, 1973; Burnard, 1990). Their aim is to produce a relaxed atmosphere in which learning can take place and a further gain is that they encourage group participation and the learning of names. They are used by many facilitators in the experiential learning field. However some people (including the author), feel more comfortable with a more straightforward form of introduction. The argument here is that people coming to a new learning experience are already apprehensive. Many carry with them memories of past learning experiences which may or may not have been of the 'formal' sort. To introduce those people to icebreakers too early may alienate them before they start. The icebreaker, by its very unorthodoxy, may surprise and upset them. A simpler form of introductory activity is to invite each person in turn to tell the rest of the group their name, where they work and their position in the team or organization and a few details about themselves that are nothing to do with work.

It is helpful if the facilitator sets the pace for the activity by first introducing herself in this way. A precedent is thus set and the group members have some idea of both what to say and how much to say. I recall forgetting this principle when running a learning session in The Netherlands. As a result, each group member talked for about ten minutes apiece and what was intended as a short introductory activity turned into a lengthy exercise! The golden rule, perhaps, is keep the activity short and sharp and keep the atmosphere light and easy-going.

Once group members have begun to get to know each other, the facilitator should deal with 'domestic' issues regarding the group's life. These will include the following.

- When the group will break for refreshments and meal breaks and when it will end.
- A discussion of the aims of the group.
- A discussion of the 'voluntary principle': that learners should decide for themselves whether or not they will take part in any activity suggested by the facilitator and that no one should feel pressurized into taking part in any activity either by the facilitator or by the power of group pressure. It is worth pointing out that if a person finds themselves alone in sitting out on a particular activity, they should not feel under any further obligation either to take part or to justify their decision not to take part.
- Issues relating to smoking in the group, when smokers are present.
- Any other issues identified either by the facilitator or by group members.

This early discussion of group 'rules' is an important part of setting the learning climate. The structure engendered by this helps everyone to feel part of the decision-making and learning process.

Identifying learning resources

In this stage, both learners and facilitator identify the resources for learning that are present within the group. This may be done with the aid of a *needs/offers* board. A large flipchart sheet or area of a black or white board is divided into two columns, 'needs' and 'offers'. Learners and facilitator(s) then fill this chart in appropriately at the beginning of a course or 'block' of learning. Clearly, this approach cannot be used at the start of the first such course or block, where neither facilitators nor learners will know each other's skills and knowledge bases. After an introductory programme, however, the needs/offers board can help determine the content of all future learning encounters.

Once both facilitator(s) and learners have written down their learning needs and what they have to offer the group, each member is then encouraged to put a tick against the items that they feel will most usefully be included in the learning period.

This approach to identifying needs and resources can be used for one-day workshops as well as for week-long study periods. It depends for its success on all members of the learning group being committed to full negotiation of content. Having said that, it would seem reasonable that the facilitator retains the right to add certain 'compulsory' topics to any given programme in line with her perception of what is required to fulfil a particular syllabus.

Planning the learning encounter

Once the learning group's needs and resources have been identified, the group can draw up a learning contract. Types of contract can range from the informally agreed list of topics used as the basis of discussion and learning during the day or week to a planned identification of what will be learned, how it will be learned and how learning will be evaluated. Such a contract will draw from the non-negotiable content drawn from the syllabus and from the wants and offers identified.

The non-negotiable content drawn from the syllabus may serve as a theme for the learning period. On the other hand, it is important that the contents drawn from the needs and offers lists are not seen as 'additions' to an already finalized timetable. The aim is not to offer learners concessions but to fully negotiate a timetable that best suits their wants and needs and yet which also fully prepares them for any examinations and practical work that they will face. The facilitator who helps in the drawing up of this initial learning contract will need to exercise considerable tact and diplomacy in handling the tension between individual and group needs on the one hand and the requirements of the syllabus on the other.

An alternative approach to using learning contracts is for each learner to draw up one for their own use. This may mean that a given group of students does not meet together for the entire period of learning but that some students will be working on their own whilst others are attending lectures, seminars, discussion and practical learning sessions.

Running the learning group

All that remains is for the learning session to progress along the lines negotiated with the group. The facilitator's task is to ensure the smooth running of the group. Variety of method is an important consideration in ensuring that all members get what they need from the learning encounter and the following represents a shortlist of methods that may be used.

- Lectures
- Facilitator-led seminars
- Student-led seminars
- Facilitator-led discussions
- Student-led discussions
- Leaderless discussions
- Experiential learning activities
- Buzz groups
- Individual learning sessions
- Demonstrations
- Visits
- Invited speakers
- Small group project work
- Small group discussion followed by large group plenary sessions

It is probably fair to say that most health-care trainers will be armed with a variety of teaching and learning strategies (but probably use only a limited number of them) whilst many learners coming to student-centred learning for the first time will tend to imagine that 'teaching and learning' necessarily involves having someone at the front of the group who leads it and does most of the talking. It is helpful if all learners coming to student-centred learning from more traditional approaches are offered a number of sessions on:

- the philosophy of student-centred learning and a rationale for its use;
- the range of teaching/learning methods that are available;
- practice in a range of teaching/learning methods and feedback on their use.

If student-centred learning is to succeed, it must involve the learners in every respect, including the skilful use of teaching and learning methods. Learning to use these methods is never wasted for they can be used again and again in future learning encounters both within educational establishments and within the clinical setting. In the clinical area, it is clearly inappropriate to use a formal 'lecture' method. It is not uncommon, however, to find mini-classrooms set up in wards and departments which exactly mimic the traditional learning approaches. The student-centred approach to learning can encourage the appropriate use of the appropriate learning aid.

Closing the group

Each facilitator will probably develop her own style of closing the group at the end of the day or at the end of a workshop. A traditional way is through summary of what the day has been about. There is an important limitation in this method. It is asserted that while the facilitator is summing up in this way, she is doing two things that are not particularly helpful. First, she is putting into her own words the experience of the group members. Second, whilst she is 'closing' in this way, group members are often, silently, closing off their thoughts about the day or the workshop in much the same way that schoolchildren begin to put their books away as soon as a teacher sums up at the end of a lesson. It may be far better to leave the session open-ended and to avoid any sort of summing up.

Alternatively, rather than allowing the day or the workshop to end rather abruptly, the facilitator may choose to use one or more of the following closing and evaluating activities.

Closing activity 1

Each person in turn makes a short statement about what they liked least about the day or about the workshop. Each person in turn then makes a short statement about what they liked most. No one has to justify what they say for their statement is taken as a personal evaluation of their feelings and experience.

Closing activity 2

Each person in turn makes a short statement about three things that they feel they have learned during the day or the workshop. This may or may not be followed by a discussion on the day's learning.

Closing activity 3

The group has an 'unfinished business' session. Group members are encouraged to share any comments they may have about the day or the workshop, of either a positive or negative nature. The rationale for this activity is that such sharing helps to avoid bottled-up feelings and increases a sense of group cohesion.

These, then, are the stages of a typical student-centred learning session and they may be adapted to suit the particular needs of the group and of the facilitator. The final part of the learning encounter may also involve checking through the group's learning contract to see whether various aspects have been covered in sufficient depth and whether changes need to be made to that contract.

FACILITATOR STYLE

Every facilitator needs to make decisions about what to do when working with a particular learning group. What she does in the group may be called her style. Clearly, facilitator styles will vary from person to person according to variables including previous group experience, teacher training, knowledge and skill levels, personal preferences, personal value systems and personal beliefs about the nature of education. However, it is useful if the facilitator (and particularly one new to facilitation) can consider what decisions she needs to make about her style before starting.

Heron (1977) suggests six dimensions of facilitator style that can help in such decision making.

Directive	Non-directive
Interpretative	Non-interpretative
Confronting	Non-confronting
Cathartic	Non-cathartic
Structuring	Unstructuring
Disclosing	Non-disclosing

The facilitator who uses the directive–non-directive dimension will make decisions about how much she intervenes in the development process of the group. At one end of the dimension, the facilitator may decide to control group discussion almost completely, by asking questions of the group but also by maintaining overall control of what happens in the group. At the other end, the facilitator will maintain a lower profile and little or no control over what happens in the group, preferring the learners to decide on the way the group develops. Whilst the non-directive end of the dimension is more student centred, there are clearly times when facilitator intervention will enable the group to move on and develop further. The skilled facilitator can make appropriate decisions about when to be directive and when to remain in the background.

The interpretative–non-interpretative dimension is concerned with the degree to which the facilitator offers explanations for what happens in the group. Interpretations of group processes can be made from a number of different points of view including, at least, the following: psychodynamic, sociological, trans-actional analytical, transpersonal and political. The facilitator who uses inter-pretation to help the learners make sense of what is happening in the group offers a theoretical framework for the learners to work with. The facilitator who offers no interpretation allows the learners to make their own decisions about what is happening and allows them to construct and develop their own theories. The problem with a non-interpretative style of group leadership is that some groups will neither notice group processes developing nor will they construct theories to account for what happens.

The next dimension is concerned with the degree to which the facilitator confronts the group at any given time in the group's development. At one end of the dimension, the facilitator is very challenging and draws attention to illogicalities and inconsistencies in group arguments. At the other end, she sits back and allows members of the group to challenge group debate. Again, as with the other dimensions, it is probably useful if the facilitator can learn to be appropriately confronting and appropriately passive, according to circumstances.

The cathartic–non-cathartic dimension refers to the amount of emotional release that the facilitator allows or seeks in a learning group. It is arguable that during the process of learning counselling and group skills it is helpful if group participants are allowed to express their feelings as part of the experiential learning process. Sometimes, too, arguments and discussions can be sharpened if participants are allowed to express strong feeling. At other times, however, it is more appropriate that emotional release does not become part of the group process. In a clinical teaching session, for example, or during a ward round it may not be appropriate for learners to express their feelings directly but that emotion could be expressed later during a student–facilitator discussion.

There are specific skills involved in helping people to express emotion. Heron (1977) argues that in the UK we have developed a 'non-cathartic society', where the norm generally is to bottle up rather than express emotion. He suggests various methods for helping groups to release pent-up emotion and courses in developing cathartic skills are frequently offered by colleges and extramural departments of universities.

Emotional release is part of the human condition. It is also frequently part of the experience of being a patient. If learners never have the opportunity to explore their own feelings then, arguably, they will be less well prepared for handling the emotional release of their patients. This is not to advocate frequent therapy or encounter groups as part of the educational experience but to acknowledge the need for health-care facilitators to enable the development of cathartic skills at some point in the health professional education programme.

The structuring–unstructuring dimension is vital in terms of student-centred health professional education. The highly structuring facilitator will organize the timetable, decide upon content, carry through the lessons and evaluate the whole procedure. In other words, the structuring facilitator is not particularly student centred. On the other hand, the learning sessions of a facilitator who is totally unstructuring may be an educational 'free for all', with little coherence or development. Again, the answer seems to lie in a sense of balance and an ability to decide when to offer structure to a group and when to allow the group to develop its own.

Heron's final dimension is the disclosing–non-disclosing one. The disclosing facilitator is one who shares with learners much of her own thoughts and feelings, as they emerge. In this sense, she becomes a fellow traveller with the learners. Many years ago, Sidney Jourard (1964) suggested that 'disclosure begets disclosure'. The facilitator who is able to share something of herself with her learners is more likely to encourage them to share something of themselves with the group. Thus the process of education becomes a humanizing process.

On the other hand, there are times when non-disclosure is appropriate. If the facilitator is too disclosing, she may find that she inhibits group participants. Most of us have experienced the person who, at the drop of a hat, tells us his life story or who too readily discloses his own thoughts or feelings. Almost as important as whether or not we disclose to a group is the decision about when we disclose. As with most things in life, timing is of the utmost importance. Sometimes to hold back and keep our thoughts and feelings to ourselves can encourage quieter members of the group to develop the courage to disclose.

The six dimensions of facilitator style have wide application across many different sorts of learning groups. Facilitators may use them in seminar groups, in organizing discussions, in running support groups and in running learning groups in clinical settings. The dimensions may also be offered to learners as a framework for considering their own decisions about running groups. Whenever we engage in a learning encounter, we make certain decisions about how to proceed. The dimensions of facilitator style offered here allow for clearcut prior decisions to be made. They also allow for 'fine tuning' whilst the group is in progress. The person who has internalized and understood the range of possibilities contained within the six dimensions can quickly change tack whilst working within a group and yet do it with some precision.

INFORMATION GIVING: MORE FORMAL TEACHING

There are, of course, times when health professionals are called upon to give lectures, hold formal teaching sessions or pass on information to others in a more formal, structured way. While the idea of facilitation is important, it is also useful to develop more traditional skills in teaching. This, then, is the 'teacher-centred' end of the scale.

The initial need is for a *framework* for thinking about formal teaching. A familiar curriculum model contains the following stages.

1. Aims of the learning encounter
2. Content of the learning encounter
3. Teaching/learning methods
4. Assessment of learning and evaluation of the encounter

Formal teaching takes preparation. Normally, someone undertaking a teaching session will prepare notes based around the aims of the session. The first question here is: Who identifies the aims of the learning encounter? At least three answers are possible.

1. The teacher
2. The students
3. The teacher and the students together

Traditionally, teachers always identified learning aims and objectives. Since the development of student-centred learning, we have seen an increasing move toward students having at least some say in what they are taught. This is based on the adult learning theory that suggests that, as adults, we are able to identify our own learning needs. In a sense, this is true in everyday life. These days, if I want to learn about something, I plan my own learning. For example, I have just learned to use a new program for analysing qualitative research data. I did not sign up to take classes in the topic but, instead, worked with the program, bought a couple of books about the program and read the manual from cover to cover. In the end, too, I will use the program as best suits me. This, then, is an example of adult learning – admittedly of the informal sort – in which the learner tacitly identifies his own learning goals. My goal was to learn to use the program to the level that allowed me to analyse interview transcripts.

Once aims have been set, the notes for the session have to be prepared. Most teachers try to teach too much. If you are new to lecturing or teaching, it is worth working out a teaching plan. Such a plan acts as an *aide-mémoire* to the teacher and helps them to plan the session. Figure 10.1 shows an example of such a teaching plan.

A teaching plan forces you to think about how much time a particular topic will take to cover. Clearly, the amount of discussion any given group will want or need varies but such a plan can usefully serve as a *statement of intent*. It also enables you to judge the ratio of 'teacher talk' to 'student talk'. It is usually more educational if the amount of student talk exceeds the amount of teacher talk although this, again, will vary from topic to topic.

ASSESSMENT AND EVALUATION

These two words are sometimes used as synonyms. As a rule, though, you *assess* students and *evaluate* courses or teaching sessions. Thus, the assessment processes that might be used in relation to the above teaching session might involve asking the students to write an essay about using counselling skills in health-care situations. Alternatively, they might involve setting a short examination.

The evaluation of the teaching session might take place at the close of the session or at the end of a term or block of teaching encounters. There are pros and cons for both approaches. It is always difficult to know *what* is being evaluated at the end of a teaching session. Often, the students are merely asked whether or not they *enjoyed* the session. It is difficult to see how they could place a value on the session before they have applied the learning from it to the 'real world'. On the other hand, if sessions are evaluated some time after they occur, it seems reasonable to assume that students will have forgotten a great deal of what the session was like (although, hopefully, they might not have forgotten the *content*). A useful compromise is to invite students at the beginning of a teaching session to

Name: James Smith
Title of teaching session: Introduction to Counselling
Group: 1st year diploma students
No of students: 30
Room: A45
Date and time: 2.30 pm, 12.5.96
Materials required: Handouts: (1) counselling skills, (2) reference list for further reading on the topic. Both × 31 copies.

Time	Activity	Topic
2.30	Talking	Introduction to definitions of counselling
2.45	Discussion	The application of counselling skills in health-care
3.00	Talking through handout	Basic counselling skills
3.15	Experiential activities	Trying out simple counselling skills, in pairs
3.45	Plenary discussion	Discussion about and evaluation of the counselling skills exercises
4.15	Talking	Summary of main points and giving out of reference list to further reading
4.30	Talking	Close session

Figure 10.1 Teaching plan.

comment on the *previous* one. In this way, too, previous learning is linked to new learning. A simple questionnaire can be devised to help in the evaluation of formal teaching sessions and the following is an example.

University of Westminster
Health-care Studies Department
Introduction to Counselling Skills

I would be grateful if you could indicate your reactions to the following statements by circling the appropriate phrase. Please respond to each of the items and circle only one item for each. Thank you for your co-operation.

James Smith

1. The aims of the session were clearly stated.
Strongly disagree   Disagree   Don't know   Agree   Strongly agree

2. The content of the session was appropriate in level.
Strongly disagree   Disagree   Don't know   Agree   Strongly agree

3. I feel that I will be able to use the content of this session in my everyday work.
Strongly disagree   Disagree   Don't know   Agree   Strongly agree

4. The session was about the right length.
Strongly disagree   Disagree   Don't know   Agree   Strongly agree

5. There was an appropriate balance between discussion and lecturing.
Strongly disagree   Disagree   Don't know   Agree   Strongly agree

6. I was encouraged to ask questions.
Strongly disagree   Disagree   Don't know   Agree   Strongly agree

7. The handouts were well prepared and will be useful to me.
Strongly disagree   Disagree   Don't know   Agree   Strongly agree

8. Overall, I felt that the session was useful and worthwhile.
Strongly disagree   Disagree   Don't know   Agree   Strongly agree

Any other comments:

SUMMARY

This chapter has taken a broad view of the process of learning through experience. All health-care professionals are concerned with learning, both their own and their colleagues'. The issues and skills that have been discussed here are relevant to *all* communication skills in the health-care professions.

References

Boud, D. and Pascoe, J. (1978) *Experiential Learning: Developments in Australian Post-Secondary Education*, Australian Consortium on Experiential Education, Sydney, Australia.

Burnard, P. (1990) *Learning Human Skills: An Experiential Guide for Nurses*, 2nd edn, Heinemann, Oxford.

Dewey, J. (1916) *Democracy and Education*, Free Press, London.

Dewey, J. (1938) *Experience and Education*, Collier Macmillan, London.

FEU (1983) *Curriculum Opportunity: A Map of Experiential Learning in Entry Requirements to Higher and Further Education Award Bearing Courses*, Further Education Unit, London.

Heron, J. (1973) *Experiential Training Techniques*, Human Potential Research Project, University of Surrey, Guildford, Surrey.

Heron, J. (1977) *Dimensions of Facilitator Style*, Human Potential Research Project, University of Surrey, Guildford, Surrey.

Jourard, S. (1964) *The Transparent Self*, Van Nostrand, New Jersey.

Keeton, M. and Associates (1976) *Experiential Learning*, Jossey-Bass, San Francisco, California,

King, E.C. (1984) *Affective Education in Nursing: A Guide to Teaching and Assessment*, Aspen, Maryland.

Knowles, M.S. (1975) *Self-Directed Learning*, Cambridge, New York.

Knowles, M.S. (1980) *The Modern Practice of Adult Education: From Pedagogy to Andragogy*, 2nd edn, Follett, Chicago.

Kolb, D. (1984) *Experiential Learning*, Prentice-Hall, Englewood Cliffs, New Jersey.

Peters, R.S. (1969) *The Ethics of Education*, Allen & Unwin, London.

Pfeiffer, J.W. and Goodstein, L.D. (1982) *The 1982 Annual for Facilitators, Trainers and Consultants*, University Associates, San Diego, California.

Rogers, C.R. (1972) The facilitation of significant learning, in *The Psychology of Open Teaching and Learning*, (eds M.L. Silberman, J.S. Allender and J.M. Yanoff), Little, Brown, Boston.

<table>
<tr><td>

11

</td><td>

Presentation skills

</td></tr>
</table>

AIMS OF THE CHAPTER

The following skills are discussed.

- Planning a presentation
- Using notes and visual aids
- Speaking
- Taking questions

Have you ever been asked to talk about your work? Many health professionals have. Once over the feeling of being flattered and having their self-confidence boosted, many go on to worry about how they will cope. This is especially true if they are asked to talk at a conference. Saying 'yes' to a request is the easy part. The more difficult bits are preparing what you have to say and then saying it. In this chapter, the whole process of preparing and giving a presentation is explored.

One thing needs to be clear. Giving a presentation at a meeting or a conference is different from teaching. First of all, the aims are different. The main aim of teaching is to enable and encourage learning. The main aim of a presentation is to offer a clear outline of some particular information. In the process of giving that information, the presenter may be teaching too but that is not the main aim.

People go to conferences and presentations to hear very specific information. Often, they are not beginners in a particular field; rather, they are co-professionals. On the other hand, it is important to remember that one of the reasons you have been asked to make a presentation is that you have information that others do not. You are the expert amongst experts. This can be an exhilarating thought but it can also be a little worrying. What can help here is *structure*: structure in planning, delivery and follow-up. In the following sections, each of these elements is examined.

PLANNING THE PRESENTATION

First, be clear. Why have you been asked to give a presentation? Is it because you are well known and they just want you at the conference because you are 'you'? If so, it often doesn't matter what your topic is. Indeed, you may be allowed to talk about a topic of your choice. Far more likely, though, is that you have been asked to address a particular set of issues or to report some research findings. First, find out the reason for being asked and be clear about the topic. Find out, too, how long you will be expected to talk for, how long you have for questions and whether the session will be chaired. If it is, you will be introduced to your audience. If not, you will have to think about how you want to introduce yourself.

Second, to whom will you be talking? To fellow professionals? To a group of learners? If so, at what point in their training or education is that group? What comes before and after your presentation? Also, how many people will be present? Whilst there is little difference in making a presentation to 100 or 400, there are important differences between talking to five or 50 people. You need to know in advance how large or small your audience will be.

What will you tell your audience? It is important that you avoid trying to include 'everything' in your presentation. If you are presenting research findings, the important things are the findings themselves. You do not need to go into elaborate background detail, nor (usually) do you need to talk a great deal about sampling procedures. From the audience's point of view, the interesting things are usually what you found in your research.

Your presentation of findings must be interesting. Bear in mind that you have lived with your work. You have found it fascinating. The task now is to inspire others. You can do that if you carefully plan your presentation.

The stages in a presentation, whatever the topic, can be divided up thus.

- Introduction (of self and topic)
- Outline of points to be covered
- Development of each of the points
- Summary and brief discussion
- Inviting questions

Think carefully about the points that you want to make and don't make too many. Most of us are familiar with the groan that occurs when someone stands up with a prepared flipchart sheet which identifies ten points and it is all too clear that the speaker is going to cover each in some detail. Try to summarize your work under three or four main headings. Then, as the audience has a signposting system through your talk and you have a scaffolding upon which to build your talk, no one is going to feel overwhelmed.

Once you have identified your three or four main points, think about how you will introduce the whole talk and how you make it obvious why you want to talk about points you raise. Remember that your aim is to *inform*. If you have done your research, you will have a reasonable idea of the 'level' of your audience.

Once this is established it will usually become clear that you do not have to offer a wide-ranging historical introduction to your subject area. Instead, all you need to do is to put your talk into context and wade into your main points.

Think carefully about timing. Whilst this obviously comes with experience of talking, you must try to work out exactly how much you can cover in the time available to you. It is very easy to overestimate how much you can say in a given time. If you stick to the 'three or four points' rule, you are less likely to overrun. Underrunning can also be a problem, although it is far less important. First, most people are quite happy to sit through a short presentation. Second, you are quite likely to be able to make up time through the question period. It can be argued that the question session is often the most valuable part. On the other hand, if people have come some distance to hear you talk, they may be disappointed if you reach your conclusion ten minutes after standing up.

One way to judge your timing is to role play your whole presentation with a colleague, a group of colleagues or members of the family. By far the most difficult option (but probably the most useful) is the second one. If you can gather together a group of colleagues to listen and make comments on your proposed presentation, you can learn a lot about how to do it and how to ensure that you neither over- or underrun. Ask those who listen to you to pay particular attention to the following.

- The way you start your presentation
- How you look as you deliver it
- Your tone of voice and speed of delivery
- Your use of language and jargon
- The way you close your presentation

Listen carefully to what your colleagues or family have to say. This is not always easy. I remember the night before I gave my first paper at an international conference, I was told by a colleague that 'It is a pity you can't do something about your monotonous voice!'. I did do something, but I can't guarantee it was the right thing. Throughout the presentation I tried to modulate my voice and probably sounded fairly bizarre. The point here is to do the role playing well in advance of your presentation. If they can bear it, have your colleagues listen to you a second time. Be careful, though, that you do not 'wear out' your talk or overrehearse it. Whilst everyone likes a polished performance, no one likes to get the impression that this is the 14th time you have given it.

NOTES

To read from notes or not? Not. If at all possible, avoid reading directly from a script or straight from notes. If you can read what you have to say, so can your audience. If all you are doing is reading what you would normally publish in a journal, do the latter. Go away and write your journal paper. Whilst you may not want to do without notes altogether (and few do), you should try to limit your notes to key issues and an overall outline structure.

The most frequently used method of using notes at a presentation is holding a bunch of index cards in your hand, each of which contains notes linked to one of your three or four points. These have advantages and disadvantages. The advantages are that they are easy to hold and to refer to. You can hold your hands up fairly high and this tends to encourage you to speak out to your audience rather than down to your notes. On the other hand, small cards can be dropped. Once dropped, you have the unenviable (but fascinating to the audience in a morbid sort of way) task of picking them up and rearranging them. Just in case, it is best to number your cards with fairly large numbers so that your nervous hands can reorder them in a crisis.

It is usually best to link your cards with your visual presentations. As noted in the next section, backing up what you say with things that the audience can look at pays distinct dividends. Usually, you can link one card with one visual aid. In this way, you do not have to carry out too many operations at once. Be sure, though, to clearly number both your cards *and* your visual aids. Visual aids can also be dropped or get out of order. If both the card and the aid bear the same number, you are less likely to run into problems.

The alternative to cards is to use a typewritten or computer-generated set of notes. If you use this method, you need to have them typed with double spacing, so that you can read them easily as you glance down. Also, it is useful to make full use of coloured 'outlining' pens. Careful colour coding can show you where you are in relation to your main three or four points: each point can be outlined in a different colour and that colour code can be carried through to your visual aids. The big disadvantage of typed sheets is that you are likely to get carried away with looking at them.

There is some comfort to be had from holding a large bunch of papers. Often, that comfort takes over and the speaker stares down at them throughout the presentation, sometimes for fear of losing their place. Think, too, about whether or not you staple the sheets together. The advantage of this approach is that you can hold the whole set of pages together, with less fear of dropping them. On the other hand, if you find yourself with a large lectern in front of you, unstapled sheets can more easily be turned over. I have been known to adopt the 'belt and braces' approach and take two sets of notes with me to a conference: one stapled and the other not.

If your confidence really leaves you and you decide that you *must* read from notes, consider the way that you write out those notes. Rather than just typing out a 'script', write out what you say in the way that you say it. The following extract illustrates this. The piece is laid out in such a way that it makes it very clear where you pause and where you take a breath. The idea is that each line contains one phrase. Work carefully through your notes and break them up in this way. This will save you 'fluffing' lines or having to re-read what you have said. It must be stressed, however, that reading direct from a paper is the last resort. If you can, avoid it.

Example of the layout of a paper to be read

Many managers are having to think carefully about how change is affecting their organization.

Many are experiencing anxiety about the *rate* of change.

Writers on the topic are not particularly helpful here.

All seem to stress that change is accelerating.

This morning, I want to challenge that view.

The question is:

Is the rate of change *really* increasing?

Think about your own work place.

What changes have *you* seen?

Major ones?

Or have you experienced a slow trickle of minor changes?

One of the best ways of preparing this sort of paper is on a computer, using a word processor. It is possible, in some programs, to set up macros or shorthand routines that operate 'sentence-busting' functions. Such macros split the whole of your paper up into sentences and put each sentence on a separate line. WordPerfect does this. With this word processor, it is possible not only to sentence-bust but also to reverse the process and put the paper back together again. In this way, you can prepare the paper that you use for your presentation and copies of it for wider distribution. Be careful, though: splitting the paper into sentences is not all that is involved. You also need to go through the piece and underline or accent certain words so that you know exactly when to emphasize your points. Notice, too, that the piece above is not strictly grammatical. You may want to consider the use of rhetorical questions that 'sound' right when you speak but would not normally be acceptable in a written paper. Again, this is further fuel for the argument that you should try to avoid reading directly from a script. On the other hand, if you are giving a lot of very detailed information which must be exactly right, then reading may be your only option. Consider, for example, newsreaders on the television. No one would expect them to extemporize with the help of cue cards.

VISUAL AIDS

Back up what you say with a visual aid. Almost all presentations can be more interesting if they are also offered visually. On the other hand, be wary of overusing such aids. If too many are used, the audience can become distracted by waiting to see what else happens in your 'performance' and they lose track of what you are saying.

Why use visual aids at all? A number of important reasons can be identified.

- Some people absorb information far more easily in a visual mode than they do in an aural one.
- The visual aid adds interest to what you are saying.
- Some things can *only* be conveyed visually (imagine trying to *say* what a magnified snowflake looks like).
- A visual aid takes attention off the speaker and allows them to breathe more easily.
- People like them.

The key issues that apply to all visual aids are keep them simple and uncluttered and keep them few in number. First, it is important that visual presentations do not contain hundreds of words and that the audience do not have to spend the next five minutes reading. Remember that all the time the audience is reading your visual aid, they are not listening to you. This means that some of your presentation will be lost and your audience may be unable or unwilling to catch up. Second, nothing is more daunting than the realization that a speaker has 20 visual aids to work through. Keep them short and keep them few in number. Finally, remember that once a visual aid has been used, it is important to remove it from view.

Four main types of visual aids for presentations can be identified.

- Overhead transparencies
- Flip charts
- Slides
- Video tapes

Overhead transparencies are probably known to everyone who has been involved in teaching or learning. They are fairly easy to prepare and can quickly convey a lot of information. What is not always appreciated is how they should be prepared. It is not uncommon to see handwritten transparencies. Far better are those prepared with a graphics package on a computer. This is as true for transparencies that contain only words as it is for those which are pictorial. Both sorts can first be drawn or typed using a program such as *Harvard Graphics* or *Applause*. Once the detail has been produced with such a program, the results can be printed out onto paper and then transferred to the acetate sheet via a photocopier. The result is nearly always more professional than with a handwritten or hand-drawn sheet. If such graphics programs are not available, another approach is to type words onto paper, enlarge the output with a photocopier and then transfer the enlarged images onto the acetate. As a rule, the less that is contained on an acetate sheet, the better. Do not type line after line. Instead, either use a series of sheets or depend upon one or two pithy lines. Figure 11.1. illustrates an example of what may go onto a single sheet. As a rule, simplicity is the keynote in overhead projector sheets. Coloured sheets may be used to add interest or to differentiate between different issues but, again, be careful. It is easy to find that your audience is more interested in *son et lumière* than in what you have to say.

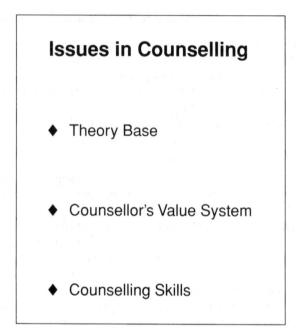

Figure 11.1 Example of a prepared overhead acetate sheet.

The flipchart sheet has become popular over the last ten years. These are giant 'drawing pads' on which the presenter either has prepared sheets of information or on which they write during the presentation. Bear in mind that many people associate their use with small group work in which participants 'brainstorm' ideas onto such sheets. The very presence of a flipchart pad and easel may have some of the audience (perhaps already anxious about what is to follow) ready to break into groups to work with their colleagues.

Rules about the preparation of acetate sheets also apply to the preparation of flipchart presentations. Because a flipchart pad is so large, it is always tempting to overfill each sheet. Resist this. Keep to a minimalist message, as was the case with acetate sheets. The items listed in Figure 11.1 could easily be transferred to a flipchart pad, without addition of other material.

Flipchart sheets must necessarily be hand drawn (although, in extreme circumstances, it may be possible to use Letraset or similar graphical lettering products). However, they have one big advantage over overhead projector sheets. The bulb in an overhead projector is a fragile thing. Murphy's law dictates that the bulb will blow just as you come to your first acetate sheet and when you are feeling at your most vulnerable. If you are nervous of this happening and you are not talking to a very large group, you may choose to use a flipchart.

If you prepare your sheets before the conference, consider leaving the first white sheet of the pad blank. Then, you need only 'disclose' what is written on each of your sheets once you have started talking. If you are allowed free use of the pad, you may want to leave a blank sheet between written sheets too. In this way, you can take a break between each of the sheets, rather in the way that you might turn the overhead projector off between acetates.

If you are going to write on the pad as you talk, be sure that your writing is neat enough to be read. It does not have to be particularly large. Usually, letters of about 1.5″ in height can easily be read by most of a medium-sized audience. Resist the temptation to 'doodle' on the pad or to write down unconnected words or diagrams. Write neatly and clearly and express only one or two ideas on each sheet. If you need to, you can tear off each sheet and 'Bluetack' it up on a wall. This does, however, take confidence. If you are nervous, it is very easy to flamboyantly rip straight through the middle of your sheet as you tear it off.

An alternative to the flipchart is the traditional black or (less traditional) white-board. Both have fallen into disuse as aids during presentations and conferences, perhaps because of their 'classroom' connotations. If you do use either of them, practise first. Both take experience to use effectively. It is easy, for instance, to find yourself talking *to* a whiteboard. It is also easy to break chalk. Finally, it is not uncommon for both chalk and whiteboard pens to run out at a critical moment. Perhaps, after all, it is for these reasons that such visual aids are rarely seen today.

Slides are yet another way of displaying parts of a presentation graphically. Whilst they are easily the most interesting format of all of the visual aids mentioned so far, they also have a variety of drawbacks. First, they are expensive to produce and difficult to produce well. It is not sufficient to be a keen amateur if you want to produce really effective slides. If you do use slides, have them professionally produced.

Another drawback to the use of slides is that so much can (and often does) go wrong. First, the slide projector can break down, either before or during your presentation. Second, because of nerves, it is very easy to put slides in to the slide carousel upside down or in the wrong order. This is usually guarded against if you have slides professionally made for presentation as the 'right side up' is usually marked on each slide. This does not, however, stop you putting them into the carousel in the wrong order. Also, if you show slides, you usually have to dim the lights. This takes the spotlight off you (which you may think is a good thing). On the other hand, once you are out of the limelight, the audience may forget you and pay more attention to your slides, becoming impatient to see the next one.

Having said all that, well-produced slide packages can easily outshine all other forms of visual aid for impact on the audience. Even slides with lettering on (used in place of overhead projector acetates) add an air of authority to the presentation. Graphs, bar charts and histograms always look more professional if they are shown on slides. The usual rule applies, though: put very little on each slide. This may be slightly more expensive but it is much better than presenting slides covered in words, figures or images.

Think carefully about the visual aids that you choose. Try to go to other people's presentations and see what worked best for them. Then choose your own aids. You may want to use more than one sort of aid: slides and a flipchart, for example. Do avoid too much visual razzmatazz: as noted earlier, it is possible for the audience to become so impressed with the 'show' that they stop paying attention to you or your presentation.

SPEAKING

When you are speaking to an audience, you want to communicate with as many members of it as possible. Certain straightforward rules apply here. First, be careful about your posture. Stand up straight, try not to wander around in front of the audience and keep an eye on your breathing. It is useful to begin the whole presentation by taking one or two deep breaths before you start. This nearly always seems to you as though you are standing silent for about 15 minutes. For the audience, however, it is a chance to really focus their thoughts on you and to settle down in their seats.

A common error when speaking in public is to focus eye contact and attention on one person. This may be due to some well-meaning but often misconstrued advice that you should 'find someone in the audience and speak to them'. Pay attention to your eye contact. Try to make regular 'sweeps' of the audience, punctuated by picking out various members of the assembly to address certain parts of your talk to. Avoid looking down at your notes as much as possible. It is here that having cards, rather than a typed script, can really pay off. The fact that you only have a small card in your hand means that your eye is not so easily drawn to it.

Be careful of the hand gestures that you make. It is easy to get carried away and forget that your hands are 'talking for you'. Make gestures mean something. If necessary (and this is difficult) practise some gestures in front of a mirror or in front of a colleague. Notice what works and what does not. Watch commentators on the television and see what gestures they use. Watch politicians, too, for they are masters and mistresses of effective gesture; at least, they are if they are good.

Finally, be aware of all aspects of your voice. Important here are the tone, volume and pitch. It is not recommended that you try to change your accent if you are not happy with it but you can practise developing the *tone* of your voice. As a general rule, the more relaxed you are, the more likely it is that your tone will be deeper and more full. If you are very nervous, your voice is likely to become 'thinner'. Again, remember the deep breaths just before you start and if you get very nervous, practise some deep breathing before your whole presentation.

Check the *volume* of your voice before you start. One way of doing this is to arrive a little early and ask someone to sit at the back of the room. Then ask them if they can hear you clearly. If you cannot do this, it is sometimes helpful to ask, at the beginning of your presentation, if everyone can hear you, especially at the back. The problem with this approach is that even if people can hear you, they are sometimes loath to call out the fact.

Prior role play can help you assess the best pitch of your voice. Is your voice naturally mellifluous or do you tend to drone a little? If you are prone to monotony in your speaking, practise a few changes of tone and add a few 'ups and downs'. In this respect, you will have to become a little like an actor. Indeed, it could be argued that part of being an effective speaker is being able to act the part. If you *look* and *sound* the part, you probably *are* the part.

TAKING QUESTIONS

Once you have given your talk or presentation, there will often be a space for you to take questions. If the conference or talk is being chaired, the chairperson will deal with questions from the floor. If not, you have to manage them yourself. It is helpful (and gives you a little time to adjust to the person asking the question) if you suggest that each person introduces themselves by name and occupation before they ask their question. This gives you a little more control over your audience. After all, there are lots of them and only one of you. If there are lots of requests to ask questions, indicate (and remember) who you will take questions from. For example, you may say: 'I'll take the lady at the back's question first and then one from the gentleman on the right'. Do keep track. People don't like to feel that they have been left out. Also, limit questions initially to one per person. This not only spreads out the questions, but it also saves your becoming embroiled in detailed discussions with one person. Particularly, look out for the following 'danger' questions.

- Questions that seek to show you up. If you have one of these, there are at least two ways of dealing with it. First, you answer it as best you can and say 'Does that deal with your point?' or you deflect the question by saying something like 'That's an interesting point; perhaps we could discuss that after the meeting'. Don't feel that you have to answer every question; listen to how politicians avoid most questions!
- Five questions rolled into one. Here, you need to be skilful at unpacking. You may want to dissect out the various issues or you may choose to answer just the first question by saying 'I think I'll just deal with the first point you raise ...'
- Questions from someone who claims to be a 'friend'. This approach is usually heralded by the person calling you by your first name and by their saying 'We talked some time ago, in York, about some of the things you have described this morning ...'. This is a particularly awkward way of being presented with a question; sometimes the question is a 'barbed' one or one that seeks to put you into a difficult light. Try not to be thrown by the 'immediate intimacy' of the questioner's approach and answer the question with a level manner. Avoid sharing the supposed intimacy. Sometimes, of course, you will suddenly be asked a question by someone that you really do know. A couple of years ago, I found myself being asked a question by a cousin that I had not seen for about

a decade. Again, here you need to take a deep breath, avoid public reminiscences and answer the question as clearly as you can.

Bear in mind that most people are 'on your side'. They are also genuinely interested in what you have to say; they would not have come if that wasn't the case. If you can, take the fact that you have been asked to speak as a compliment. Enjoy yourself if you can but don't get carried away. Keep an eye on the clock or put your watch down in front of you and stick to a firm schedule. Then, stand back and let them know that you've arrived!

SUMMARY

This chapter has examined a number of aspects of presenting your work to an audience. It has described the importance of preparation and structure. It has also discussed some of the visual aids that you may want to use to illustrate your talk. Finally, it has discussed some of the personal issues involved in the 'presentation of self'. At a conference or talk, you are selling yourself. Do it well.

12

Computing skills

AIMS OF THE CHAPTER

The following issues are discussed.

- Buying a computer
- Using a computer
- Word processing
- Spreadsheets
- Graphics
- Databases
- Using computers in research
- The Internet

You can't go far without encountering computers in one form or another. The present generations of children and students are growing up completely computer literate while older health professionals may be struggling to come to terms with using computers. Either way, many people arrive at the point where they have to decide whether or not to buy one. If they do decide to buy one, they have next to think about what sort and about what software to buy. In this chapter, we explore aspects of buying and working with home computers. Many of the issues in this chapter will also apply to computers at work, in both clinical and community settings.

BUYING A COMPUTER

Why buy a computer at all? Many people are finding that they are useful for a range of applications in the home. The most usual reason for buying one, as far as health professionals are concerned, is for completing course work towards further education or degree studies or for research work.

Other obvious applications in the health professional and home context are:

- for the preparation of teaching material;
- for keeping notes;

- for the maintenance of bibliographies and book lists;
- for doing accounts;
- for keeping address and contact lists.

What computer should you buy? Computer hardware (the keyboard, monitor and computing unit itself) is changing rapidly. It is also dropping in price. Any specific advice about particular models of computer would be out of place but certain general suggestions can be made. A computer for use in the home that is not going to age too quickly should fulfil most and perhaps all of the following criteria.

- It should be IBM compatible. IBM set a certain standard for computing equipment at the end of the 1980s. Whilst many computers are 'IBM clones' and it is not necessary to buy a genuine IBM machine, it is essential that the computer that you buy is fully compatible with IBM machines. There is a range of Apple Macintosh computers now available which are also IBM compatible. Alternatively, of course, you may prefer to use an 'exclusively' Macintosh computer but in this case it is more difficult to run programs written for IBM and IBM-compatible computers.
- It should have a hard disk. A hard (as opposed to floppy) disk is capable of storing vast amounts of data. Whilst larger capacity floppy disks are being developed, hard disks currently allow for the storage of 1–2 gigabytes of data and above. The hard disk also allows you to store all your programs inside the computer and saves you having to find disks and load up programs from 'outside'.
- It should be expandable. Many computers have 'expansion slots' inside them which allow for upgrading in line with current technological developments. Some of the cheaper and smaller ones do not. It is not necessary to keep changing hardware to keep up with every development. On the other hand, if you do not keep up with some of the main developments, you may find that you can no longer find software to work with your computer as it gets older.
- It should have a monitor and keyboard that suit you. On the monitor issue, many feel that a black and white screen is ideal for word processing. On the other hand, some feel that a colour screen gives them more flexibility. Yet others prefer a large-sized screen that allows you to see and work on a whole A4 page of print at a time. Obviously, larger screens also cost more and are 'non-standard'. Similarly, the 'feel' of a keyboard is the subject of much debate. Some prefer a keyboard that reminds them of a typewriter and 'clicks' when the keys are pressed. Others prefer a 'deader' keyboard. It is recommended that you try typing on a range of keyboards before you choose yours. This is one of the problems when buying computers through the post. Unless you have had experience of the model that you order, you will not be able to try out the keyboard before you buy.
- It should have sufficient RAM (random access memory) to allow you to use modern programs. As computers develop, so the RAM requirements grow. Until fairly recently, a computer that had 4 Mb of memory was thought to be

adequate. Now it is not uncommon to find machines with 16 Mb fitted as standard. If you cannot afford to buy a computer with a lot of RAM fitted as standard, make sure that you can expand the memory at a later date.

Where should you buy a computer? It is sometimes tempting to walk into high street branches of electrical stores and wander round their computer departments trying to decide what you should buy. This is fine if you know what you are looking for but the assistants in such shops are rarely computer experts. It is probably better to enlist the help of a computer expert at work, someone who knows about your own work and your own computing needs. Most health organizations have one or two resident computer experts so you shouldn't have to look far.

Second, become familiar with the computers that you have at work. Learn about them, their capacities and their costs. Then get to know the computer magazines and begin to compare prices. Often, buying through the post can be an excellent way of getting a good computer at a fair price. The obvious limitation is that you must know what sort of computer you want. Also, make sure that the firm that you buy it from offers you after-sales service.

Whilst most computers are fairly reliable and have relatively few moving parts to break down, it is important that you can get help on the spot when you need it. Watch out for the companies that insist on a 'back to base' warranty. This means that if your computer breaks down at home, you are responsible for returning it to the company for repair.

There is never a 'right time' to buy a computer. It seems to be a fact of life that just as you get your first computer, you realize that it is already out of date. This is just a reflection of the rapid development of the computing industry that shows no sign of levelling off. You just have to live with it.

Once you have bought your computer (or better still, before you buy it) learn to type. It is surprising how many people still use the 'hunt and peck' approach to the keyboard and continue to type with two fingers. Part of developing keyboard skills is learning to type. Two approaches are possible here. On the one hand it is practical to attend evening classes in typing or a weekend intensive workshop. On the other hand, there are now many software packages that allow you to develop typing skills at the keyboard. Such programs offer a graded and timed approach to learning how to type and are a cost-effective and time-economical way of advancing keyboard skills.

USING A COMPUTER

Get into the habit of working in a consistent way with your computer. If you have a hard disk, make sure that you organize your files on it in a logical way. With the large amounts of space available on such a disk, it is quite easy to lose files if you do not organize them into directories and subdirectories. The manuals that come with your computer will tell you how to do this.

The one golden rule of computing is to make frequent backups of your work, so that you always have more than one copy of every file that you work on. Then, if a file gets lost, destroyed or 'corrupted' in some way, your work has not been lost. This rule is particularly important if you have a hard disk. It is easy to believe that hard disks are reliable and not subject to breakdown. Generally, this is true. The point is, though, that hard disks have a finite life. At some point, they all *do* break down. If this happens and you have not made backups of your work, your work is lost. Make backups of all the writing that you do and of any new data files that you work on. If, for example, you add references to your bibliographic database (see below), make sure that you backup the database onto another disk.

WORD PROCESSING

The word processor is probably the most frequently used program in any home or office computer. Essentially, it allows you to edit and re-edit your work without having to retype everything that you have written. Compare this with typewriting. If you use a typewriter and make a mistake, you have to use a correction paper or fluid and risk making a mess of the paper or you retype the whole page.

With a word processor, neither of these options is necessary. If you make a mistake, if you want to reorder paragraphs or change the text completely, you merely go back to the screen and make the changes. Only when you are completely happy with what you have written do you print out your final 'hard' copy. Word processors vary immensely in their complexity. As with all things, you tend to get what you pay for as the more fully featured programs tend to be very expensive. Check before you buy one that you need all the features on offer and you will be able to learn how to use it fairly easily. Like other skills, word processing taking practice. It's not like sitting down at a typewriter and beginning to type. With a word-processing program you need to invest some time in learning how to use it. Such learning is repaid by cleaner pages, better organized work and the knowledge that you are no longer frightened of computers. Some of the important features to look for in a word processor are:

- the ability to move text easily;
- a spell-checking routine;
- a feature for word counting;
- the ability to work with more than one document at once;
- the ability to insert page numbers.

As you become more proficient at word processing you may want to move up to a more comprehensive program, especially if you do a lot of business, academic or creative writing. Other, more advanced features include:

- an indexing facility;
- the ability to work with graphics, diagrams and boxes;

* a thesaurus facility;
* a function for pulling together a number of files;
* macros or the ability to enter a string of commands with a single key stroke.

SPREADSHEETS

A spreadsheet program allows you to develop a huge 'rows and columns' chart to undertake a whole range of calculations on all or on a selection of the rows and columns. In some ways it is like a computerized and automated accounts book. On the other hand, it can also do far more than just compute rows and columns. It can be used for at least the following functions too.

* Storing addresses
* Compiling bibliographies and reference lists
* Drawing 'word illustrations' in column format.

GRAPHICS

Graphics packages allow you to illustrate and generally 'dress up' your work. A top commercial package will help you to do the following.

* Generate graphs, histograms and pie charts
* Use 'clip art' to illustrate newsletters and projects
* Make slide presentations
* Generate charts for use as overhead projections in teaching
* Draw organization charts

A good graphics program can make your work look more professional and can help you to communicate your thoughts through iconic representation. A basic rule applies here, though: keep it simple. Graphics programs can generate very complicated illustrations and diagrams and it is easy to get carried away with what they can do. Generally communication is much clearer if you stick to simple charts and representations.

DATABASES

After the word processor, the database program is probably one of the most useful for the student, teacher and practitioner in the health professions. Essentially, a database program helps you to store information in a readily retrievable format. The obvious use of a database in this context is for storing references and bibliographies. Databases can also be used for storing other sorts of information from simple name and address lists through to patient records. Clearly, if the latter are being kept, it is important to ensure that you comply with the Data Protection Act. Database programs will usually allow you to:

- index your information in various ways;
- print reports of selected information;
- transfer information from the database to other programs;
- allow 'mail-merging' or the generation of multiple letters addressed to different people.

Again, the keyword is simplicity. Commercial database programs are very powerful and often quite difficult to learn to use. If your aim is to keep track of a number of bibliographies, try one of the simpler database programs. Alternatively, you may decide merely to keep your bibliographies as files within your word processor. There are a number of advantages to this approach. First, you can very readily transfer information from the data file to the one you are working in. Second, you do not have to close down one program in order to access your lists of references. Third, you do not have to learn another program. On the other hand, a database program will be much faster and much more versatile if you have bibliographies that run into hundreds of references. I used a file in my word processor to list all my references until the number reached about 500. Then I switched to using a database for them and found the increase in speed and accessibility paid off considerably.

Some people never use databases for storing references and prefer to stick to a card file. The argument is usually that it is just as quick to flip through a box of cards for a reference as it is to start up the computer and fire up the database program. This is fine if the card file is not too big. The point about a database program is that it can let you make 'selective' searches of your references and print them out. For example, you can pull out all the references that you have on counselling or all those by a particular author *and* about a specific topic. It can show you all the papers written on a particular topic after or before a certain date and so on.

COMMERCIAL SOFTWARE

Commercial software refers to the programs that are sold on the open market and produced by software companies. Many of the best known programs are very expensive to buy. On the other hand, they are nearly always very reliable and trustworthy. They also come with very detailed handbooks about their use. If you buy commercial software, only you are allowed to use it. You cannot make copies of it for your colleagues and friends.

The example of a book is a useful one here. You can *lend* someone your book, just as you can allow someone else to use your computer. What you must not do is to photocopy that book. Commercial software usually works on a similar principle. Once you have bought a program, it must only be used by one person at as DOS) and, if you use it, *Windows*. It is essential, for example, to know how to save files to disk, how to backup files, how to find them again and how to check the functioning of the hard disk. It is also important to be able to do some 'first aid' when things go wrong.

Basic training in using hardware can be organized in various ways. First, larger colleges of nursing will often have their own internal computer departments. These in turn will often employ teachers and trainers who can respond to particular needs of students and lecturers. It is advisable for anyone who is new to computing to attend an 'introduction to computers' course, which may run over one or more days.

Those who do not have access to in-house hardware training can often attend evening classes at local colleges. Most now have introductory courses and many also offer training courses in the use of specific software.

Software training also comes in various forms. First, it is possible to train yourself. Almost all software now comes with excellent manuals. On buying or using a new piece of software it is essential to sit down and read the first part of the first manual. Most of these manuals take the reader right the way through the essentials of working with a particular program, from turning on the computer through starting up the program to working with its essential features. Most programs also have built-in 'help' screens, often triggered by pressing the F1 button at the top of the keyboard. For the person who finds self-instruction difficult, there are now numerous, commercially published handbooks about specific programs available from most bookshops.

Software training is also available in colleges either in the form of short work-shops and study days or as a series of evening classes. More expensive but often more helpful are workshops organized either by the software companies themselves or by 'approved' training centres. These often have limits on the numbers of participants who can attend and usually offer a great deal of 'one-to-one' attention.

Often, learning one program means that others are easier to learn. A number of companies make interlinking 'suites' of programs. Microsoft, for example, publish a software suite known as *Office* which contains a state-of-the-art word processor, a spreadsheet and a graphics package. All these programs work in a similar way and once you have learned one of them, you can usually use the others.

Computing skills, like all other skills, require practice. It is important to set aside some time each week to learn a little more about a program. It is a sad fact that most word-processor users only use about 20% of a program's functions. Learning a little more about a program can, in the longer term, save time and produce better-looking documents.

In summary, it is important to know about the hardware as well as the programs that are used on any given computer. Second, learning about particular programs can take place 'in-house', through colleges or through attending special training centres. Finally, as with most things, it is possible to be an independent learner. If you take this path, you may have some sticky moments and may have to rescue yourself from some tricky situations but, on the other hand, you will learn a great deal.

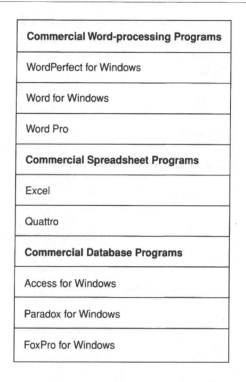

Commercial Word-processing Programs
WordPerfect for Windows
Word for Windows
Word Pro
Commercial Spreadsheet Programs
Excel
Quattro
Commercial Database Programs
Access for Windows
Paradox for Windows
FoxPro for Windows

Figure 12.1 Examples of commercial software programs.

a time and copies must not be made for distribution to others. The only exception to this general rule is that most companies allow you to make a backup copy of the program in case the original disks get damaged. Figure 12.1 offers examples of some commercial programs.

SHAREWARE

Shareware has a unique marketing strategy. A shareware program is distributed free of charge (although a charge is usually made for the disks and the handling). The idea is that you first try the program and then, if you like it, you send away a registration fee to use the program. In the first instance, you usually have between 30 and 90 days to try out the program before you register it. Further, during this time, you are encouraged to make copies of the program for your colleagues and friends. Then, the same principles apply: they are allowed to try out the program and then send off to become registered users if they find it useful.

The advantages of the shareware approach are many for the home PC user. First, you get a chance to try the program before making a financial commitment to it. Second, the registration fees for shareware are considerably cheaper than

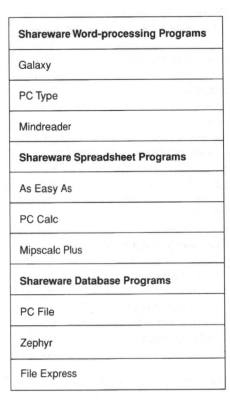

Shareware Word-processing Programs
Galaxy
PC Type
Mindreader
Shareware Spreadsheet Programs
As Easy As
PC Calc
Mipscalc Plus
Shareware Database Programs
PC File
Zephyr
File Express

Figure 12.2 Examples of shareware software programs.

copies of most commercial programs. Also, the quality of shareware programs is improving all the time and some of the best are easily the equal of commercial software. Finally, shareware offers you the easy approach to learning more about computer programs and exploring a variety of methods of working with data that you may not have been able to afford if you had to rely on buying commercial packages. Figure 12.2 illustrates some of the shareware programs that are available. The names and addresses of shareware distributors are available in any of the monthly computer magazines. Such magazines often include one or two shareware programs on a 'free' disk attached to the front cover.

Shareware is not free. The idea, as we noted above, is to try out the program, decide if you like it and then pay for it. If you decide not to use the program then you simply give the disks to another person or format the disks for use with other files. The only free programs are those available in the public domain. These public domain programs are often distributed by the same people that handle shareware although it is often not made clear in their catalogues what is shareware and what is public domain.

There are various others programs available that are useful to the health professional. Some of them are commercial programs but a good many are available as shareware. A shortlist of these other types of software would include:

- statistical packages;
- personal organizers and diaries;
- accounting packages;
- computer-aided drawing programs;
- desktop publishing programs;
- educational programs;
- aids to learning about computing;
- programs that allow you to communicate with other computers.

As your knowledge and use of computers increase and as computing equipment becomes cheaper, you may want to consider buying a modem. A modem allows you to send computer files down a standard telephone line to another computer. It also allows you to contact other computer users through 'bulletin boards' or computerized message stations. A considerable amount of shareware is available through this means and also some public domain or free software.

A modem can also aid communication between home and office. You may choose, for example, to work at home on certain days and to send in your work via the modem. This is of particular value to those who engage in writing reports and printed matter.

COMPUTER AND SOFTWARE TRAINING

First, it is important to distinguish between two types of training: training in the use of the hardware and training in the use of the software. Hardware is the computer, printer and any other 'add-on' equipment. Software is the programs that are run on the computer. Any regular user of computers needs to have some knowledge of both. From a hardware point of view, it is important to know how to turn on and start the computer. It is important, too, to be able to set up the printer to work properly. Given the general usefulness of computers it is odd to report that getting a printer to work can be one of the more difficult parts of computing.

From the software point of view, it is necessary to know how to use certain basic programs. Most scholars and researchers will need to use a word processor for the production of essays, reports, dissertations and articles. Many people use word processors as glorified (and, often, less than glorified) typewriters. This misses the point. A word processor is far more than just a sophisticated typewriter and it can change the way that you work with textual documents. Training, is essential although, as we shall see, this can be 'self-training'.

Other health-care professionals may want to use spreadsheets, graphics packages, databases and statistics packages. In a more general way, though, it is important to know how to work with the basic operating system (usually

THE INTERNET

To access the Internet is to communicate on a global level. The Internet is a giant network of computers and network of networks. It can be accessed by anyone who has a fast computer, a fast modem and the appropriate Internet connection. A modem links your computer to a phone line and enables your computer to read and write to the Internet. Finally, the Internet connection is via the phone line to a local 'provider', a company that enables you to link up to the Internet. Once connected, your only phone costs are normally those to your provider. In other words, even though you have international access to other computers and a whole host of services, you only pay the costs of being on the phone to the local provider. For this facility, you pay the local provider a monthly fee, which at the time of writing varies between £6 and £12. Figure 12.3 offers some details of service providers in the UK.

BBC Networking Club: Telephone 0181 576 7799

CityScape: Telephone 01223 566950

CIX (Computerlink Information Exchange): Telephone 0181 390 8446

CompuServe: Telephone 0800 289 458

Delphi Internet: Telephone 0171 757 7080

Demon: Telephone 0181 371 1000

The Direct Connection: Telephone 0181 317 0100

Easynet: Telephone 0171 209 0990

Eunet GB: Telephone 01227 266466

Genesis Project: Telephone 01232 231622/231719

GreenNet: Telephone 0171 713 1941

Lunatech Research: Telephone 01734 791900

Pavilion Internet Plc: Telephone 01273 607072

PC User Group: Telephone 0181 863 1191

Pipex: Telephone 01223 250120

Poptel: Telephone 0171 249 2948

RedNet: Telephone 01494 513 333

Total Connectivity Providers: Telephone 01703 393392

U-NET Ltd: Telephone 01925 633144

Figure 12.3 Some UK Internet providers.

If you work in a university or college, it is likely that you will have access to the Internet through the local college network. Increasingly, too, there are local cafés which provide access to the Internet via a computer while you eat and drink. If you have to organize your own Internet connection, the two important issues are having the fastest computer you can with the largest amount of memory and having a fast modem. *Computer Shopper* (1996) offers the following tips about buying a modem.

1. Make sure your phone systems can cope with having a modem connected. If you are plugging directly into a phone line, this will mean checking the number of equipment items already on the line. If you are plugging into a phone system you will need to check with the supplier for compatibility.
2. Look for a modem with a baud rate of at least 14 400. Anything less is outdated; anything more should cut your phone bills.
3. Internal card modems are the most reliable solution for regular modem access, such as a daily call-out. Portable modems are more flexible but often more expensive.
4. Where possible, go for a BT-approved modem, although you can save money opting for a non-approved one if you can get a recommendation.
5. ISDN is the preferred solution for regular exchange of high volumes of data. Note that both the sending and receiving ends of this connection need to be equipped with an ISDN line.

Why bother with the Internet?

Simply because it can be so useful. Although the phrase 'surfing the Internet' conjures up something done in private by socially inadequate individuals sometimes referred to as 'anoraks', there is no doubt that there is a vast amount of information on the Internet and it offers a useful and extremely quick way of communicating with others. You might use it, for example, for any one of the following (and this is necessarily a short list; the Internet is growing daily, even hourly).

1. To write to colleagues, friends, clients all over the world and have them reply quickly and easily. This happens via e-mail (or 'electronic mail'). E-mail is probably the most widely used of the Internet functions.
2. To join newsgroups and to enter into debates with other people on any topic that interests you. There are numerous medical and health-related newsgroups and they can help you to keep up to date.
3. To find new bibliographical references, search the libraries of universities and institutions in other countries (and other languages).
4. To access a huge number of encyclopaedias and other reference works or even to read whole books (the complete works of Shakespeare and huge numbers of novels are available, complete, on the Internet).

5. To access wide ranges of computer software. There are huge libraries of shareware on the Internet that are easily found and downloaded onto your computer although, if you do this, you *must* institute some form of virus checking before you download. Also, shareware has to be paid for if you decide to keep using it.
6. To keep up with the news in almost any country, in many languages and to follow events as they occur.
7. To watch video clips, explore exhibitions in art galleries, look through cameras many thousands of miles away.
8. To access the WorldWide Web, a huge collection of pages of information, graphics and music, all interconnected to other pages.

The Internet is huge and growing all the time. In 1995 Bride reported as follows.

In early Spring 1995, there are over 4.8 million host computers supplying services and information over the Net, and the number of users is estimated to be anything from 20 to 50 million. By the time you read this, those figures will be out of date, for the rate of growth is phenomenal. The number of host computers has doubled every year for the last four years, and there is plenty of scope for future expansion.

E-mail

Electronic mail is the feature of the Internet that most people use. To send e-mail messages, you need your own e-mail address (which will be issued to you by your Internet provider), the appropriate software to send and receive e-mail, the setup outlined above for access to the Internet and other people's e-mail addresses. An e-mail address is a short string of letters and characters which look something like this: HammondPT@samnet.ac.uk. The 'HammondPT' part of the address identifies the person (although many people use aliases or even numbers as this part of their address). The 'samnet' part of the address identifies the Internet access provider. The 'ac' identifies that the address is from an academic institution and the 'uk' indicates that the user is based in the United Kingdom.

To send an e-mail message, you simply enter the other person's address, type the message, press a button marked 'Send' and the message is on its way. It may travel via a huge range of other computers to get to its destination and may take anywhere from a few seconds to half a day to arrive. If it does *not* arrive, then you will be notified of this on your computer screen.

Once someone has e-mailed you you will have their address and can easily reply to their message. Incoming e-mail messages can be stored and this allows you to build up an e-mail address book. Oddly enough, finding people's e-mail address is not always that easy. As yet, there is no definitive e-mail directory. Often, the easiest way of finding someone's e-mail address is, ironically, to phone them up and ask them. Many people and many companies, too, include their e-mail address as part of their printed address on notepaper.

E-mail communication has many advantages over other sorts of communication although these take a little while to appreciate if you are new to the system. First, the system is probably the fastest way of ensuring that a message is delivered and answered. Second, it is very easy to use and does not involve typing a letter, printing it and posting it or faxing it. You simply type your message at the keyboard, press a button and send your message. It is particularly useful for keeping in contact with people in other countries. Where there is a considerable time difference between the two countries, you can send your message in the afternoon and almost guarantee a reply in the morning. Negroponte (1995) notes the nature of e-mail style as a form of communication.

> ... today, with computer ubiquity, the advantages of e-mail are overwhelming, as evidenced by its skyrocketing use. Beyond the digital benefits, e-mail is a more conversational medium. While it is not spoken dialogue, it is much closer to speaking than writing. ... I always look at my e-mail first thing in the morning and later in the day I am capable of saying 'Yes, I spoke to so-and-so this morning', whereas it was only e-mail.

Another big advantage of e-mail over other forms of communication is that you can choose when you respond to e-mail messages. Phone calls 'have' to be answered whereas you can decide in which order you respond to your e-mail messages and even decide not to answer some of them. Further, unlike telephone calls, the messages are recorded and a file full of e-mail messages can act as a 'history' of your communication pattern over a year. You might develop such a history through careful filing of letters but e-mail allows this history to be developed automatically.

Finally, perhaps for many the most important value of the e-mail system is that you can attach *computer files* to messages. Let us imagine, for example, that you are a researcher in the health-care field and want to co-write a journal paper with another researcher in another country. You type up your draft of the paper in your word processor and save the file. You can then 'attach' that file to an e-mail message and send it to your colleague who then opens your file, works on it in their word processor and returns it to you via e-mail. This sort of facility makes co-operative research between people in different countries considerably easier than if hard copies of documents have to be posted or faxed between countries. The important thing, too, is that all *codes* and *formatting* instructions remain intact when files are e-mailed in this way. It is quite possible, for example, to send a spreadsheet file and have a colleague somewhere else in the world work on the figures in it and return it to you.

Overall, e-mail represents a considerable communication advantage over ordinary mail (sometimes referred to as 'snail mail') and over the fax. It can be argued, too, that it is an improvement over the telephone. E-mail documents can be printed out, filed, referred to again, commented on, written on and treated in all the ways that any other printed document can be treated. On the other hand, a phone call is ephemeral and, usually, not recorded.

There is one rather odd feature of e-mail that needs to be observed: humour does not necessarily travel very well across it. What appears to be a witty or funny remark to the sender can quite easily be misinterpreted by the reader. Exactly why this is the case is not clear but misunderstandings in this area can cause 'flaming' – angry replies being sent to e-mail messages. I suspect that some potentially useful relationships have been spoiled unintentionally by the ill-considered use of humour. This is not to say that all e-mail communication should be without it but simply to note that you may want to exercise judgement in this area before you write anything that you consider comical. Luoto (1996) is instructive on these points.

> Once we start exchanging e-mail with strangers, over broader contexts, especially those that touch on issues which are dear to our hearts and beliefs, where the parties may come from different fields, backgrounds, or cultures, where the usage of words is not standardized or well-defined, including abstract nominalizations, then we should not be at all surprised that misunderstandings and escalating emotions abound.
>
> I'll go out on a limb and make a prediction. I think that over time, as people become more familiar with the medium of e-mail, and with how it operates, its limitations, including this known phenomenon, people will adjust and learn to take extra care as they read e-mail to give a triple-dose of benefit-of-the-doubt to others when they feel that twinge of emotion. They might learn to supply a warm, loving internal voice, perhaps that of a trusted friend, to recite the message for them as they read it, especially if it's from a stranger.

There are certain conventions based on practicality and economy that should be observed in e-mail writing. Downloading e-mail messages can take time and can cost money. Therefore, it is reasonable to observe the following.

1. Keep your e-mail messages short. Reserve your long thoughts for letters.
2. Respond to e-mail messages promptly. Many *Windows*-based e-mail programs allow you to be 'prompted' when an e-mail message arrives. It is often hard not to respond to these prompts.
3. If you use a 'signature' attached to the bottom of your outgoing e-mail messages, keep it short. Many people like to have their name and address appearing at the ends of their messages. It is probably not a good idea, though, to include your phone number in such a signature. Remember that e-mail goes to all sorts of people. You may or may not want them ringing you up.

The WorldWide Web

The WorldWide Web is a giant, worldwide collection of millions of computerized printed pages. Within the pages are *hyperlinks* or highlighted words which can be clicked on with the left-hand mouse button. This causes another page to appear on the screen, related to that word. In turn, that page will have other highlighted words that act as links to other pages and so on. In this way, it is possible to reference and crossreference items as you read them. This is also the way that many people get round the Internet, by clicking and opening different pages through the hyperlink words. Access to the WorldWide Web is achieved most easily via a Web viewer. At the time of writing, the most popular of these is *Netscape* but software for navigating the Web is developing all the time, as is the Web itself. Web pages can be downloaded to disk or printed out. Once you have found a particular page, you can mark it with a *bookmark* that allows you to return to that page, directly, at another time. You may then use the Web browser in two different ways. First, you can collect and mark useful pages. Then you can read those pages or print some of them – or sections of them – out. This process is not dissimilar to literature searching in a library: first you find the papers and collect them together and then you sit and read them through.

It takes some self-discipline to limit yourself during a web-surfing session. It is easy to get drawn into working around the various pages and the process is not dissimilar to thinking itself. You find that pages about one topic lead you to pages about others. These, in turn, point you to very different sorts of topics. It is easy to be distracted by what is on the screen and by what you read. Also, this sort of surfing can take you down blind alleys. Fortunately, there are various ways of searching the Web pages for particular items or topics. All the Web browsers offer such a search facility and there are various other search engines available on the Internet. Most people, it seems, learn about the Internet by working with it interactively. And just as you begin to believe that you have some idea of its size, you suddenly find other huge areas of information that you did not know were there. The sheer volume and diversity of information available on the Internet and in the Web pages can be overwhelming.

All Web pages have their own 'address'. One way of finding a particular page is simply to type that address into your Web browsing program. Here are some examples of 'sites' that you may want to visit via the Internet. Each address contains one or more pages of information. In many cases, huge numbers of pages are involved and, as we have seen, the pages are linked and interlinked in various ways.

All the following addresses should be prefixed with *http://* although this is inserted by default by most of the up-to-date browsers.

Educational Texts
Site address:www. etext.org/
This is an archive containing hundreds of thousands of book texts ranging from the complete works of Shakespeare to obscure scripts of past TV programmes.

Electronic Journals
Site address:
www.cern.ch:80/hypertext/DataSources/bySubject/Electronic_Journals.html
This WorldWide Web Virtual Library listing of magazines and periodicals

available on the Internet provides links to either the full text or details of the publication. Type addresses like this very carefully!

Elsevier Science
Site address: www.elsevier.nl
Elsevier claim to be the leading suppliers of scientific information. This site contains a comprehensive listing of journals, other publications, reviews and information about multimedia products.

Online Bookshop
Site address: www.bookshop.co.uk/
This site claims to be the largest online bookstore in the world with over 750 000 titles available from huge numbers of publishers.

Medscape
Site address: www.scp.com
This is a medical forum for all health professionals and contains huge amounts of medical information.

UK Internet Lists
Site address: www.limitless.co./uk/inetuk/
This is a very useful listing of available UK Internet resources. It includes lists of Internet providers, consultants, training courses, information, guides and publications about the Internet. An essential site to visit if you are new to the Internet and just as useful if you are not.

It is important to remember that the Internet is organic and changing and enlarging all the time. Some sites (and the above is only a very brief glimpse of what is available) become extinct, new ones are introduced and others are enlarged and developed. At the time of writing, a very useful resource for working with the Internet is Angus Kennedy's *The Internet and WorldWide Web: The Rough Guide*, published by Penguin. It has the advantages of being very competitively priced, small in format and very readable. Once you get into the Internet, though, there is a huge amount of information within it to help you navigate and find what you want.

USING COMPUTERS IN HEALTH-CARE RESEARCH

More and more health-care professionals are required to do research. Some are professional researchers or academics. Others have to do small-scale research projects as part of degree or higher degree programmes. The computer has changed the way in which research is conducted. This section considers some of the computers and computer methods that can be used in the process of doing research.

The palmtop computer

Many health-care professionals are now computer literate. Many are familiar with using a desktop or notebook computer and the software that goes with it. Many are also being asked to complete research projects, either as part of a degree or diploma programme or as funded projects (Burnard and Morrison, 1994). This section looks at a compact method of collecting data in health-care research projects. The method can be used to keep notes, fill in questionnaire items and even to produce interview transcripts. It can also be used to *analyse* and *interpret* the data obtained (Riley, 1990).

Many health-care research projects require that data are collected in the field (Burgess, 1984). The field, in the case, is often the clinical or the community setting and the ideal tool is a small computer which can be kept handy but which is unobtrusive. The Psion Series 3A *palmtop* computer is considerably smaller than a notebook computer. It is extremely portable and runs on two AA batteries for up to 40–60 hours, although a mains transformer is also available. In order to make full use of this computer in research settings, you also need a linking cable to enable data files to be transferred to a desktop or notebook personal computer and the program *WinLink* to facilitate that data movement. Below, the computer is described, along with the two accessories indicated above. Then, various applications in health-care research are identified.

The Psion Series 3A is a tiny hand-held computer that is smaller than a Filofax or desk diary. It contains a miniature but full and standard keyboard. While it is not really possible to touch type on the keyboard, you can achieve a reasonable speed in typing and data input is not a problem. By way of example, this chapter was written on a Series 3A.

Data are stored either in the computer's internal memory or on insertable 'flash' or RAM cards. Using these cards, the full capacity of the machine can be increased to 2 megabytes. Even the standard memory of the computer – 512K – is sufficient to store significant amounts of data. The computer has in-built software applications, including a database program, a word processor, a spreadsheet and a personal organizer. The personal organizer can contain attached 'memo' files and these are useful for keeping dated field notes (Burnard, 1995). There are other features that may be of value to the researcher including a method of organizing alarms and a means of tracking time in any part of the world. When the computer is switched off, all data contained in it are automatically stored. A lithium 'backup' battery ensures that data are never lost even if the two AA batteries run flat. Thus, all programs and data are, initially at least, held in the memory of the computer. This means that the computer has no disk drive of any sort, no hard drive and no moving parts.

The linking cable can be used to 'pipe' files into a personal computer for use with a more standard word processor. Thus a series of field notes or interview transcripts could be piped over to a PC to enable data analysis. Similar transfers can be made from all applications. The program *WinLink* works with *Windows* and enables quick and easy transfer of files through the cable. The standard cable comes with its own software but *WinLink* makes the transfer process much easier.

The Series 3A can be carried anywhere and can easily be put in a handbag or briefcase or even a pocket. This means that the researcher can have it with them at all times so data are always available and a means of recording notes and interviews is always at hand. We turn now to specific applications.

First, the research plan has to be drawn up and aims and objectives identified. Then, data collection methods need to be decided upon (Fink and Kosecoff, 1985; Crabtree and Miller, 1992). Once these have been identified, it can be decided whether or not the Series 3A could be useful. The following sections identify how each of the computer's software applications might be used in various research projects.

First, the database program can be easily tailored to suit the specific needs of a project. For example, a database could be opened in which each 'form' in the database identifies a series of questionnaire items. The researcher, having identified a member of their sample, then turns on the machine, opens the database, asks the questions and records the answers. The database will hold as many sets of answers to the questions as are required by the project. The format of the database is such that different sorts of answers to different questions can quickly be found and even added up. Thus 'frequency counts' are quite easily achieved with the database.

Second, the word-processing program can be used to transcribe interviews. This can be achieved 'live' if necessary. In this case, the researcher (who would have to be able to type fairly quickly) would transcribe the interview as it happened. While it would not normally be possible to record every word spoken, the skilled researcher could easily take detailed notes of the interview. As we have seen, the word-processing files could then be transferred to a personal computer for further analysis.

The spreadsheet program can also be used for the collection and analysis of numerical data. Thus, once the questionnaire items in the database have been completed, the findings from the questionnaire can be collated, transferred to the spreadsheet and a variety of simple, descriptive statistics computed. The findings can then be illustrated in the form of bar charts, another facility offered by the spreadsheet program.

Alongside the use of the database, word processor and spreadsheet applications, the researcher can keep a 'research diary' by using the personal organizer. This feature contains a diary which can be viewed in a day, week, month or year format. As we have seen, it can also contain lengthy 'memos' which can be attached to any day or date. With the personal organizer, the researcher can keep a record of interviews, applications of the questionnaire or any other dates in the research calendar. They can also keep short or lengthy field notes by using the memo feature.

The data in the memory of the Series 3A can be backed up to a flash or RAM card (available as optional extras) and these can be stored away from the research sites so that at least two sets of data are always available. Most researchers have horror stories of how they lost whole data sets from their computers through not having kept a reliable set of backup disks. It is recommended that data is backed up at least twice. Thus one flash or RAM card could be kept in the computer at all times while another one is stored in another location.

Data can be transferred over to a personal computer using the link cable at regular intervals, perhaps at the end of a working day in the field. *WinLink* enables the word-processing files from the Series 3A to be converted to *WordPerfect* format. This can be 'read' by a range of standard word-processing programs, including *WordPerfect* itself, *Word for Windows* and *WordPro*. There is also a facility for transferring files as simple 'text' files. These can also be read by most word processors. Transfer of information can take place in both directions. The skilled user will be able to work on data in a word processor in a desktop computer and then transfer them to the Series 3A by way of the link cable.

In this way, the Series 3A can be used in any of the following types of health-care research programmes.

- Clinical or educational surveys using questionnaires (Oppenheim, 1992)
- Semistructured or structured interview projects (Brenner, 1985)
- Evaluations of clinical practice and health care (Abrahams, 1984)
- Educational research projects in which students and/or teachers are interviewed (Davis, 1987)
- Projects in which 'baseline' data are collected (McNeil, 1990)
- Projects in which data from existing records are utilized (Sommer and Sommer, 1991)
- Longitudinal studies in which varieties of numerical and/or textual data are collected (Treece and Treece, 1986)

As we have seen, the computer can be used to store data and to analyse it in various ways.

There is increasing pressure on clinicians and academics to do research. Any methods and equipment that can help in the process of collecting and analysing data should be welcomed. Also, the number of stages in the research process should be reduced, if possible. Given that many health-care professionals can already use personal computers, the use of the Series 3A is a simple step. It is compact enough to be used in a wide range of situations. It will also run for many hours without needing a change of batteries and movement of data between it and other computers is straightforward. It is an ideal instrument for both the beginner and the experienced health-care professional researcher in a variety of quantitative and qualitative studies.

The equipment described in this section could also be used in much larger research projects. A team of research assistants, for example, could easily learn to use the Series 3A and work with identical questionnaires or interview schedules that could be programmed into a set of machines. The Series 3A also comes complete with a programming language that will be familiar to those who have experience of Basic or C.

Using a database to manage structured interview data

Interviews are widely used as a data collection method in qualitative research projects (Brenner 1985; Fink and Kosekoff, 1985; Miles and Huberman, 1994). Interviews have to be transcribed and they can generate a substantial amount of text (Krippendorf, 1980; Field and Morse, 1985). This section offers a method of managing the textual data from structured interviews. Increasingly, health-care professionals are conducting interview surveys as part of diploma, graduate and postgraduate studies (Morse, 1991; Butterworth, 1991) .

In structured interviews each respondent is asked the same sorts of questions (Sommer and Sommer, 1991). As an example, a structured interview protocol for a project in which respondents were interviewed about reflective practice might contain the following questions.

1. How would you define the term 'reflective practice'?
2. What do you feel are the advantages of a reflective practice approach in health care?
3. What do you feel are the disadvantages of a reflective practice approach in health care?

Each respondent would be asked these questions (and, presumably, a number of others). The issue then arises as to how best to manage the data that arise out of these interviews. The interviewer normally needs a method of drawing together all the responses to question 1, question 2, question 3 and so on. It is at this stage that the database program can be used.

The term 'database' can be used to describe any structured collection of information. A set of cards containing details of bibliographical references is a database as is any set of questionnaire responses. The term is used here to describe a particular type of computer program which helps the user to structure, store, find and analyse data.

Examples of commercially available database programs for the personal computer include *Access, Dataease, Paradox* and many others. Nearly all database programs involve the use of three concepts: the *table*, the *form* and the *report*. All three are useful to the researcher using structured interviews as a data collection method.

The *table* is a large grid that contains all the data in a database. It is usually made up of a series of rows and columns. Thus, the rows may represent the interview respondents and the columns their responses to each question (see Figure 12.4).

The *form* serves a number of purposes. First, it can be used to *enter* data into the database. A simple form would prompt the user to enter data, one respondent at a time. This is illustrated in Figure 12.5. Second, it can be used for *viewing* data in the database. If the researcher wanted to look at all the respondents' responses to question 3, the form would be the means by which this would be achieved. The form also allows the researcher to do *searches* on the data. In this way, they may check how often the expression 'reflective practice' is mentioned by respondents.

	Question 1	Question 2	Question 3
	How would you define the term 'reflective practice'?	What do you feel are the advantages of a reflective practice approach?	What do you feel are the disadvantages?
Respondent 1			
Respondent 2			
Respondent 3			

Figure 12.4 An example of a table.

Name	
Response to question 1	
Response to question 2	
Response to question 3	

Figure 12.5 An example of a form for data entry.

The *report* feature is self-explanatory: it is the means by which various subsets of the data can be printed out. If the researcher wanted to print out all the responses of one respondent, they would use the report feature. They might also use it to print out all the responses to particular questions.

Armed with these three tools, the researcher has the means of storing interview transcripts, finding particular transcripts, breaking down the interviews into separate questions and finding subsets of data from all the transcripts. All this needs a little planning and this is usually best done with a pad and pen. The best database layouts are usually achieved by drawing, freehand, a sketch of the sort of database structure that is required.

The researcher who uses the same questions for each interview will normally set up the database with a table of the type illustrated in Figure 12.4. If each line represents one respondent, then each column represents one of the questions asked. This simple breakdown of the data means that, later, the researcher will be able to pull out various subsets of the data and perform a highly structured *content analysis* (Krippendorf, 1980; Carney, 1982; Crabtree and Miller, 1992).

Various types of form will be needed. First, there will have to be a form for *entering* the data and a template for this is illustrated in Figure 12.5. This shows a simple format in which one form is used for each respondent and in that form is typed each of that respondent's responses to the questions. The database program automatically transfers this information into the table. At a later date, this information can be taken out of the table via a second series of forms.

The second series of forms will involve those that draw together all respondents' responses to each question. Thus, the first form in this series will relate to question 1. The form will display each respondent's response to that question. This can then be printed out as a report or saved in the computer. In this way, each of the forms in the series draws together all of the responses to each of the questions in a highly structured way (see Figure 12.6). The information grouped together in this way can later be transferred to a word processor for preparation of the research report.

Various other considerations have to be made. First, the researcher needs to be sure about the layout of the data entry forms at the beginning of the project. Thus, if the interview schedule is to have ten questions, then the form must contain ten fields for data entry. Also, the researcher has to assess the likely length of each response and allow sufficient space in each entry field to accommodate the responses. With many databases, it is not easy to change the structure after data entry has begun. The researcher therefore needs to do a series of trial runs of data entry to iron out any possible difficulties with data entry, data storage or data retrieval. If it

Question 1 [respondent 1]	Reflection involves thinking about what you do, as you do it. It's sort of important to remember to reflect. You can't just expect to be able to do it.
Question 1 [respondent 2]	There are various forms of reflection, I suppose. The way I would use it would be to stop after doing something and spend some time thinking about all the aspects of what I have just done. I'm not sure that this is the only way of defining it.
Question 1 [respondent 3]	Reflection ... it's really what everyone does. You have to do it. You probably couldn't get by if you didn't. I don't know, really ...

Figure 12.6 An example of a form used to draw together all responses to a question from structured interviews.

is anticipated that responses to questions are likely to be lengthy, then the field *types* should be set to 'memo'. Normally, fields in a database have a limit to the amount of data that can be entered into them; sometimes this is as little as 250 characters. *Memo fields*, however, allow substantial amounts of text to be entered.

Also, the researcher must be prepared to transcribe interviews directly into the database. The advantages of using the database program are lost if the researcher first types the transcripts into a word processor and then cuts and pastes the information into the database. The whole point of using the database is to structure the information and to economize on time so that effort can be put into other parts of the research process.

In summary, the database can be used to store, organize and offer a simple content analysis of interview transcript data. Although a database program can never *analyse* data, only *organize* it (as with all computer software), it does offer a means of handling interview data in an organized and easy-to-use manner. The method is particularly useful in projects in which large datasets are involved.

It should be noted, too, that databases can also be used for storing and analysing *numerical* data such as that generated by questionnaires. Often, though, there are more appropriate statistical programs available for this sort of work, such as *SPSS* or *SyStat*.

The method of handling data described in this section refers to *structured* interview data. Database programs are also available for handling less highly structured information and these are known as *freeform database* programs. Examples include *Idealist* and the oddly named *AskSam*. It should be noted, however, that these sorts of programs generally have less well-developed forms and reporting features. What they do allow, though, is detailed *searching*. In other words, they allow the researcher to identify recurrent words and phrases within datasets. This means that the researcher can use them for other types of content analysis such as the analysis of single words or strings of words (Berg, 1989). This is useful when the researcher wants to perform a *quantitative* analysis of textual data – when they want to ask the question 'How *many* occurrences are there of this word or phrase in my dataset?'. There are also dedicated qualitative data analysis programs available such as *The Ethnograph* and *NUD*IST*.

*NUD*IST* is a particularly flexible program that runs under *Windows*. It allows you to import textual data of various sorts and in various forms and then create whole sets of categories for analysing the text. Category sets can be created before analysis or during it. Also, the category system can be reformulated later in the project and this form of working can enable the development of *theories* from the data. The program can also help you to undertake certain forms of *quantitative* analysis and it does not depend on the researcher using a particular research approach. Thus *NUD*IST* can be used by those doing grounded theory research, ethnography, phenomenology and so on. While the handbook is not the easiest one to follow (although this may well have improved by the time this book is published), the program has an excellent tutorial attached to it and getting the hang of the program is a fairly intuitive process after a little experimentation.

Computers and computer programs are useful in a range of research situations in health-care (Sommer and Sommer, 1991; Burnard, 1995). This section has identified one way in which database programs can help the health-care professional researcher to organize their data.

SUMMARY

This chapter has considered a range of issues relating to computers as a means of communication in the health-care setting. In the end, we all have to use them. To learn about them now is an investment.

References

Abrahams, P. (1984) Evaluating soft findings: some problems of measuring informal care. *Research, Policy and Planning*, **2**(2), 1–8.

Berg, B.L. (1989) *Qualitative Research Methods for the Social Sciences*, Allyn & Bacon, New York.

Brenner, M. (1985) Intensive interviewing, in *The Research Interview: Uses and Approaches*, (eds M. Brenner, J. Brown and D. Canter), Academic Press, London.

Bride, M. (1995) *The Internet*, Hodder Headline, London.

Burgess, R. (1984) *In the Field: An Introduction to Field Research*, Unwin Hyman, London.

Burnard, P. (1995) *Health Care Computing*, Chapman & Hall, London.

Burnard, P. and Morrison, P. (1994) *Health Care Research in Action: Developing Basic Skills*, Macmillan, London.

Butterworth, A. (1991) Generating research in mental health care. *International Journal of Health Care Studies*, **28**(3), 237–46.

Carney, J. (1982) *Content Analysis*, Harper & Row, London.

Computer Shopper (1996) Shopper's guide to buying modems, April.

Crabtree, B. and Miller, W. (eds) (1992) *Doing Qualitative Research*, Sage, Beverly Hills, California.

Davis, B. (ed.) (1987) *Health Care Education: Research and Developments*, Croom Helm, London.

Field, P.A. and Morse, J. M. (1985) *Health Care Research: The Application of Qualitative Approaches*, Croom Helm, London.

Fink, A. and Kosecoff, J. (1985) *How to Conduct Surveys: A Step-By-Step Guide*, Sage, Beverly Hills, California.

Luoto, K. (1996) *Sensitivity and e-mail*. Psych-couns discussion list. Psych-couns@mailbase.ac.uk. 14.7.96.

Krippendorf, K. (1980) *Content Analysis: An Introduction to Its Methodology*, Sage, Beverly Hills, California.

McNeil, P. (1990) *Research Methods*, 2nd edn, Routledge, London.

Miles, M. B. and Huberman, A. M. (1994) *Qualitative Data Analysis*, 2nd edn, Sage, Thousand Oaks, California.

Morse, J. (ed.) (1991) *Qualitative Health Care Research: A Contemporary Dialogue*, Sage, Beverly Hills, California.

Negroponte, D. (1995) *Being Digital*, Black Arrow, London.

Oppenheim, A. (1992) *Questionnaire Design, Interviewing and Attitude Measurement*, 2nd edn, Pinter, London.

Riley, J. (1990) *Getting the Most from Your Data: a Handbook of Practical Ideas on How to Analyse Qualitative Data*, Technical and Educational Services Ltd, Bristol.

Sommer, B. and Sommer, R. (1991) *A Practical Guide to Behavioural Research: Tools and Techniques*, 3rd edn, Oxford University Press, Oxford.

Treece, E.W. and Treece, J.W. (1986) *Elements of Research in Health Care*, 4th edn, C.V. Mosby, St Louis, Missouri.

Skills check: Part Four

Sit quietly and reflect on the skills that have been discussed in this section. How many of them are applicable in your health-care setting? To what degree do you feel that you have had training in those that are applicable?

Now ask yourself the following questions.

- What do I need to do to enhance my skills in the area of education?
- How effective am I as a teacher?
- What are my presentation skills like?
- If I was asked to make a presentation tomorrow, what would I have to do now?
- Do I have the skills I need in computing?
- Do I use computers effectively?
- Could I use computers to do effective research?

Appendix:
Personal communication skills questionnaire

You can use this questionnaire in various ways.

- As a self-assessment and self-evaluation instrument before, during and after reading this book
- As a means of identifying which skills you need to work on further
- As a basis for discussion in group work

Ring the appropriate answer following each statement.

Teaching skills

1. I am quite good at learning from my own experience

Strongly agree   Agree   Don't know   Disagree   Strongly disagree

2. I am good at helping others to learn from their own experience

Strongly agree   Agree   Don't know   Disagree   Strongly disagree

3. I am better at teaching than facilitating

Strongly agree   Agree   Don't know   Disagree   Strongly disagree

4. I prefer facilitation to teaching

Strongly agree   Agree   Don't know   Disagree   Strongly disagree

5. Most of my educational experiences have been formal ones

Strongly agree   Agree   Don't know   Disagree   Strongly disagree

6. Most health professional training is teacher centred

Strongly agree   Agree   Don't know   Disagree   Strongly disagree

7. Therapy is a form of education

Strongly agree   Agree   Don't know   Disagree   Strongly disagree

Presentation skills

8. The idea of making a presentation to a group of colleagues is not a daunting one

Strongly agree   Agree   Don't know   Disagree   Strongly disagree

9. The idea of making a presentation at a conference worries me

Strongly agree   Agree   Don't know   Disagree   Strongly disagree

10. I would handle a formal presentation better than an informal one

Strongly agree   Agree   Don't know   Disagree   Strongly disagree

11. I would not be sure of my ability to produce effective visual aids

Strongly agree   Agree   Don't know   Disagree   Strongly disagree

Computing skills

12. I am computer literate

Strongly agree   Agree   Don't know   Disagree   Strongly disagree

13. I do not know how to use a computer

Strongly agree   Agree   Don't know   Disagree   Strongly disagree

14. I am happy with a word processor but not with a spreadsheet

Strongly agree   Agree   Don't know   Disagree   Strongly disagree

15. I have no use for a computer

Strongly agree   Agree   Don't know   Disagree   Strongly disagree

Listening skills

16. I am not a naturally good listener

Strongly agree   Agree   Don't know   Disagree   Strongly disagree

17. I listen to other people very well

Strongly agree   Agree   Don't know   Disagree   Strongly disagree

18. I enjoy listening to others

Strongly agree   Agree   Don't know   Disagree   Strongly disagree

19. I listen to clients well, but not so well to colleagues

Strongly agree   Agree   Don't know   Disagree   Strongly disagree

Counselling skills

20. I would like to be more effective as a counsellor

Strongly agree   Agree   Don't know   Disagree   Strongly disagree

21. I think counselling is part of every health professional's role

Strongly agree   Agree   Don't know   Disagree   Strongly disagree

22. I think counselling should be left to professionals

Strongly agree   Agree   Don't know   Disagree   Strongly disagree

23. I would like to learn the basics of counselling

Strongly agree   Agree   Don't know   Disagree   Strongly disagree

Group skills

24. I don't enjoy the prospect of running a group

Strongly agree   Agree   Don't know   Disagree   Strongly disagree

25. I enjoy being a group participant

Strongly agree   Agree   Don't know   Disagree   Strongly disagree

26. I think I would be quite effective as a small group facilitator

Strongly agree   Agree   Don't know   Disagree   Strongly disagree

27. I enjoy running groups

Strongly agree   Agree   Don't know   Disagree   Strongly disagree

Management skills

28. I manage people well

Strongly agree   Agree   Don't know   Disagree   Strongly disagree

29. I am fairly organized in my work

Strongly agree   Agree   Don't know   Disagree   Strongly disagree

30. I manage time effectively

Strongly agree   Agree   Don't know   Disagree   Strongly disagree

31. I would like to be better at managing people

Strongly agree   Agree   Don't know   Disagree   Strongly disagree

32. I would prefer to handle my time more effectively

Strongly agree   Agree   Don't know   Disagree   Strongly disagree

Meeting skills

33. I enjoy going to meetings

Strongly agree   Agree   Don't know   Disagree   Strongly disagree

34. I am quite effective as a chairperson

Strongly agree   Agree   Don't know   Disagree   Strongly disagree

35. I dread being asked to take the minutes

Strongly agree   Agree   Don't know   Disagree   Strongly disagree

36. Meetings are not really my cup of tea

Strongly agree   Agree   Don't know   Disagree   Strongly disagree

37. I think our organization has too many meetings

Strongly agree   Agree   Don't know   Disagree   Strongly disagree

Interview skills

38. I always get nervous if I am asked to do interviews

Strongly agree   Agree   Don't know   Disagree   Strongly disagree

39. I would prefer to be interviewed than to interview others

Strongly agree   Agree   Don't know   Disagree   Strongly disagree

40. I am not very organized when I interview people

Strongly agree   Agree   Don't know   Disagree   Strongly disagree

41. I am not sure how to draw up a curriculum vitae

Strongly agree   Agree   Don't know   Disagree   Strongly disagree

Writing skills

42. I could never write anything for publication

Strongly agree   Agree   Don't know   Disagree   Strongly disagree

43. I would like to see something I had written in print

Strongly agree   Agree   Don't know   Disagree   Strongly disagree

44. I could never write a book

Strongly agree   Agree   Don't know   Disagree   Strongly disagree

45. I read a lot: perhaps I could write

Strongly agree   Agree   Don't know   Disagree   Strongly disagree

46. I have always wanted to write

Strongly agree   Agree   Don't know   Disagree   Strongly disagree

Assertiveness skills

47. I don't seem to be able to say 'no' to people very easily

Strongly agree   Agree   Don't know   Disagree   Strongly disagree

48. I would prefer to be more assertive

Strongly agree   Agree   Don't know   Disagree   Strongly disagree

49. I think that people who say they are assertive usually mean that they are aggressive

Strongly agree   Agree   Don't know   Disagree   Strongly disagree

50. I am very assertive

Strongly agree   Agree   Don't know   Disagree   Strongly disagree

51. I am too assertive

Strongly agree   Agree   Don't know   Disagree   Strongly disagree

52. I'm not sure that assertiveness is very important for health professionals

Strongly agree   Agree   Don't know   Disagree   Strongly disagree

Self-awareness skills

53. Self-awareness is essential for health professionals

Strongly agree   Agree   Don't know   Disagree   Strongly disagree

54. No one is really very self-aware

Strongly agree   Agree   Don't know   Disagree   Strongly disagree

55. I think that nobody can become truly self-aware

Strongly agree   Agree   Don't know   Disagree   Strongly disagree

56. I would prefer it if I knew myself better

Strongly agree   Agree   Don't know   Disagree   Strongly disagree

57. Other people know me better than I know myself

Strongly agree   Agree   Don't know   Disagree   Strongly disagree

58. You can't teach people how to be self-aware

Strongly agree   Agree   Don't know   Disagree   Strongly disagree

59. People I know tend to be more self-aware than me

Strongly agree   Agree   Don't know   Disagree   Strongly disagree

60. Self-awareness is largely a question of learning from personal experience

Strongly agree   Agree   Don't know   Disagree   Strongly disagree

There is no formal system for scoring this questionnaire although it is possible to devise one. One method would be to allocate a value to each of the statements thus:

32. I would prefer to handle my time more effectively

Strongly agree	Agree	Don't know	Disagree	Strongly disagree
5	4	3	2	1

It should be noted that for some questions, the values should be reversed, thus:

22. I think counselling should be left to professionals

Strongly agree	Agree	Don't know	Disagree	Strongly disagree
1	2	3	4	5

Once values have been allocated in this way, according to what are considered to be 'right' answers, the scores for each statement are added together and an overall score is obtained. This system may be of value if the questionnaire is used in a group setting or as a means of checking personal progress over a period of time. The real problem with this sort of scoring is establishing which answers are the 'right' ones. It is suggested that many of your responses to questions will depend on your own situation, your own values and your own preferences. For this reason, it is recommended that the questionnaire be used as a personal or small group instrument of reflection and not adapted for use as a research instrument without further validation.

Bibliography

Abraham, C. and Shanley, E. (1992) *Social Psychology for Nurses*, Edward Arnold, London.

Adamek, M. (1994) Audio-cueing and immediate feedback to improve group leadership skills: a live supervision model. *Journal of Music Therapy*, **31**, 135–64.

Adams, N., Bell, J., Saunders, C. and Whittington, D. (1994) *Communication Skills in Physiotherapy-Patient Interactions*, Research Report, Centre for Health and Social Research, University of Ulster, Jordanstown.

Adelman, R.D., Greene, M.G., Charon, R. and Friedmann, E. (1992) The content of physician and elderly patient interaction in the medical primary care encounter. *Communication Research*, **19**, 370–80.

Allcock, N. (1992) Teaching the skills of assessment through the use of an experiential workshop. *Nurse Education Today*, **12**(4), 287–92.

Altshuler, K.Z. (1989) Will the psychotherapies yield different results? A look at assumptions in therapy trials. *American Journal of Psychotherapy*, **63**(3), 310–20.

Analoui, F. (1993) *Training and Transfer of Learning*, Avebury, Aldershot.

Anastasi, T. (1987) Communication training, in *Training and Development Handbook: A Guide to Human Resource Development*, (ed. R. Craig), McGraw-Hill, New York.

Anderson, B. and Anderson, W. (1985) Client perceptions of counselors using positive and negative self-involving statements. *Journal of Counselling Psychology*, **32**, 462–5.

Anderson, L. and Sharpe, P. (1991) Improving patient and provider communication: a synthesis and review of communication interventions. *Patient Education and Counselling*, **17**, 99–134.

Anderson, M. and Gerrard, B. (1984) A comprehensive interpersonal skills program for nurses. *Journal of Nursing Education*, **23**(8), 353–5.

Arnold, E. and Boggs, K. (1989) *Interpersonal Relationships: Professional Communication Skills for Nurses*, W.B. Saunders, Philadelphia.

Ashworth, P.D. and Longmate, M.A. (1993) Theory and practice: beyond the dichotomy. *Nurse Education Today*, **13**(5), 321–7.

Atkins, S. and Murphy, K. (1993) Critical thinking: a foundation for consumer-focused care. *Journal of Continuing Education in Nursing*, **18**(8), 1188–92.

Au, S. and Li, C. (1992) A fresh start in the East End ... Chinese counselling service. *Nursing Times*, **88**(10), 65–6.

Audit Commission (1993) *What Seems to Be the Matter? Communication between Hospitals and Patients*, HMSO, London.

Auerbach, K.G. (1991) Assisting the employed breastfeeding mother. *Breastfeeding Review*, **2**(4), 158–66.

Aune, R.K. and Kikuchi, T. (1993) Effects of language intensity similarity on perceptions of credibility, relational attributions, and persuasion. *Journal of Language and Social Psychology*, **12**, 224–37.

Bachelor, A. (1988) How clients perceive therapist empathy: a content analysis of 'received' empathy. *Psychotherapy*, **25**, 277–40.

Bailey, R. and Clarke, M. (1989) *Stress and Coping in Nursing*, Chapman & Hall, London.

Baker, S., Daniels, T. and Greeley, A. (1990) Systematic training of graduate-level counsellors: narrative and meta-analytic reviews of three major reviews. *Counselling Psychologist*, **18**, 355–421.

Baldwin, T. (1992) Effects of alternative modelling strategies on outcomes of interpersonal skills training. *Journal of Applied Psychology*, **77**, 147–54.

Baldwin, T. and Ford, K. (1988) Transfer of training: a review and directions for future research. *Personnel Psychology*, **41**, 63–105.

Baldwin, T. and Magjuka, R. (1991) Organisational training and signals of importance: effects of pre-training perceptions on intentions to transfer. *Human Resource Development*, **2**, 25–36.

Barker, J.R. and Tompkins, P.A. (1994) Identification in the self-managing organisation: characteristics of target and tenure. *Human Communication Research*, **21**, 223–40.

Barkham, M. and Shapiro, D.A. (1986) Counselor verbal response modes and experienced empathy, *Journal of Counselling Psychology*, **33** (1): 3–10.

Barkham, M., Shapiro, D.A. and Firth-Cozens, J. (1989) Personal questionnaire changes in prescriptive vs. exploratory psychotherapy. *British Journal of Clinical Psychology*, **28**, 97–107.

Barnlund, D.C. (1993) The mystification of meaning: doctor–patient encounters, in *Perspectives on Health Communication*, (eds B. Thornton and G. Kreps), Waveland Press, Illinois.

Baron, R. (1988) Negative effects of destructive criticism: impact on conflict, self-efficacy, and task preference. *Journal of Applied Psychology*, **73**, 199–207.

Baruth, L.G. (1987) *An Introduction to the Counselling Profession*, Prentice-Hall, Englewood Cliffs, New Jersey.

Batty, R., Barber, N., Moclair, A. and Shackle, D. (1993) Assertion skills for clinical pharmacists. *Pharmaceutical Journal*, **251**, 353–5.

Baum, B.E. and Gray J.J. (1992) Expert modelling, self-observation using videotape, and acquisition of basic therapy skills. *Professional Psychology: Research and Practice*, **23**, 220–5.

Bayntun, L.D. (1993) Setting the scene for experiential learning. *Nursing Standard*, **7**(36), 28–30.

Beisecker, A.E. (1990) Patient power in doctor–patient communication: What do we know? *Health Communication*, **1**, 105–22.

Bell, C. (1991) Using training aids, in *Gower Handbook of Training and Development*, (ed. J. Prior), Gower, Aldershot.

Bellack, A. and Hersen, M. (eds) (1988) *Behavior Assessment*, Pergamon, New York.

Bensing, J. and Dronkers, J. (1992) Instrumental and affective aspects of physician behaviour. *Medical Care*, **30**, 283–98.

Berger, B.A. and Felkey, B.G. (1989) A conceptual framework for focusing the teaching of communication skills on compliance gaining strategies. *American Journal of Pharmaceutical Education*, **53**, 259–65.

Bernstein, L. and Bernstein, R. (1980) *Interviewing: A Guide for Health Professionals*, 3rd edn, Appleton-Century-Crofts, New York.

Bettinghaus, E.P. and Cody, M.J. (1994) *Persuasive Communication*, 5th edn, Harcourt Brace, Orlando, Florida.

Billow, J.A. (1990) The status of undergraduate instruction in communication skills in U.S. Colleges of Pharmacy. *American Journal of Pharmaceutical Education*, **54**, 23–6.

Binder, J.L. (1993) Observations on the training of therapists in time-limited dynamic psychotherapy. *Psychotherapy*, **30**(4): 592–8.

Bird, J., Hall, A., Maguire, P. and Heavey, A. (1993) Workshops for consultations on the teaching of clinical communication skills. *Medical Education*, **27**, 181–5.

Blanck, P.D., Buck, R. and Rosenthal, R. (eds) (1986) *Nonverbal Communication in the Clinical Context*, Pennsylvania University Press.

Bland, M. and Jackson, P. (1990) *Effective Employee Communications*, Kogan Page, London.

Blenkinsopp, A., Robinson, E. and Panton, R. (1994) Do pharmacy customers remember the information given to them by the community pharmacist? in *Social Pharmacy: Innovation and Change,* (eds G. Harding, S. Nettleton and K. Taylor), The Pharmaceutical Press, London.

Blondis, M. and Jackson, B. (1982) *Nonverbal Communication with Patients*, Wiley, New York.

Board, M. and Newstrom, J. (1992) *Transfer of Training*, Addison-Wesley, Reading, Mass.

Bohart, A.C. (1988) Empathy: client-centred and psychoanalytic. *American Psychologist*, **43**, 667–8.

Bond, T. (1993) *Standards and Ethics for Counselling in Action*, Sage, London.

Bor, R. and Watts, M. (1993) Talking to patients about sexual matters. *British Journal of Nursing*, **2**(13), 657–61.

Borisoff, D. and Purdy, M. (eds) (1991) *Listening in Everyday Life*, University of America Press, Maryland.

Bostrom, R.N. (1990) *Listening Behavior*, Guilford Press, New York.

Boud, D. (ed.) (1981) *Developing Student Autonomy in Learning*, Kogan Page, London.

Boud, D., Keogh, R. and Walker, M. (1985) *Reflection: Turning Experience into Learning*, Kogan Page, London.

Bower, G.H. and Hilgard, E.R. (1981) *Theories of Learning*, 5th edn, Prentice-Hall, Englewood Cliffs, New Jersey.

Bowes, A. and Domokos, T. (1995) South Asian women and their GPs: some issues of communication. *Social Sciences and Health*, **1**, 22–34.

Bowling, A. (1991) *Measuring Health: A Review of Quality of Life Scales*, Open University Press, Milton Keynes.

Bowman, F.M., Goldberg, D.P., Millar, T. *et al.* (1992) Improving the skills of established general practitioners: the long-term benefits of group teaching. *Medical Education*, **26**, 63–8.

Boydel, E.M. and Fales, A.W. (1983) Reflective learning: key to learning from experience. *Journal of Humanistic Psychology*, **23**(2), 99–117.

Bradley, A. and Phillips, K. (1991) Interpersonal skills training, in *Gower Handbook of Training and Development*, (ed. J. Prior), Gower, Aldershot.

Brandon, D. (1991) Counselling mentally ill people. *Nursing Standard*, **6**(7): 32–3.

Brearley, S. (1990) *Patient Participation: The Literature*, Scutari Press, Harrow.

Brinko, K. (1993) The practice of giving feedback to improve teaching. *Journal of Higher Education*, **64**, 576–93.

Brookfield, S. (1993) On impostorship, cultural suicide and other dangers: how nurses learn critical thinking. *Journal of Continuing Education in Nursing*, **24**(5), 197–205.

Brosius, H. and Bathelt, A. (1994) The utility of exemplars in persuasive communications. *Communication Research*, **21**, 48–78.

Brown, D. and Srebalus, D.J. (1988) *An Introduction to the Counselling Process*, Prentice-Hall, Philadelphia.

Brown, R. (1988) *Group Processes: Dynamics Within and Between Groups*, Basil Blackwell, Oxford.

Buchan, R. (1991) An integrated model of counselling. *Senior Nurse*, **11**(4), 32–3.

Buckley, R. and Caple, J. (1990) *The Theory and Practice of Training*, Kogan Page, London.

Buckman, R. (1992) *How to Break Bad News: A Guide for Health-Care Professionals*, Macmillan, London.

Buckroyd, J. and Smith, E. (1990) Learning to help … teaching counselling. *Nursing Times*, **86**(35), 54–7.

Buetow, S. (1995) What do general practitioners and their patients want from general practice and are they receiving it? A framework. *Social Science and Medicine*, **40**, 213–21.

Buller, D.B. and Aune, R.K. (1992) The effects of vocalics and nonverbal sensitivity on compliance: further tests of the speech accommodation explanation. *Western Journal of Speech Communication*, **56**, 37–53.

Burgoon, M., Hunsaker, F. and Dawson, E. (1994) *Human Communication*, Sage, Thousand Oaks, California.

Burke, J.F. (1989) *Contemporary Approaches to Psychotherapy and Counselling: The Self-Regulation and Maturity Model*, Brooks/Cole, Pacific Grove, California.

Burley-Allen, M. (1995) *Listening: The Forgotten Skill*, Wiley, New York.

Burnard, P. (1990) So you think you need a computer? *Professional Nurse*, **6**(2), 119–20.

Burnard, P. (1991) The language of experiential learning. *Journal of Advanced Nursing*, **16**(7), 873–9.

Burnard, P. (1991) Using video as a reflective tool in interpersonal skills training. *Nurse Education Today*, **11**, 143–6.

Burnard, P. (1992) Defining experiential learning: nurse tutors' perceptions. *Nurse Education Today*, **12**, 29–36.

Burnard, P. (1992) Learning from experience: nurse tutors' and student nurses' perceptions of experiential learning: some initial findings. *International Journal of Nursing Studies*, **29**(2), 151–61.

Burnard, P. (1992) Some problems in understanding other people: analysing talk in research, counselling and psychotherapy. *Nurse Education Today*, **12**(2), 130–6.

Burnard, P. (1992) Student nurses' perceptions of experiential learning. *Nurse Education Today*, **12**(3), 163–73.

Burnard, P. (1992) *What is Counselling?* Bridge Medical Books, Houghton, Essex.

Burnard, P. (1993) Personal Computing for Health Professionals, Chapman & Hall, London.

Burnard, P. (1993) Using experiential learning methods with larger groups of students. *Nurse Education Today*, **13**, 60–5.

Burnard, P. (1994) *Counselling Skills for Health Professionals*, 2nd edn, Chapman & Hall, London.

Burnard, P. (1994) Developing the reflective practitioner: exploring new methods in nurse education. *Asian Journal of Nursing Studies*, **1**(2), 20–3.

Burnard, P. (1994) *Interpersonal Skills Training*, 2nd edn, Kogan Page, London.

Burnard, P. (1994) Searching for meaning: a method of analysing interview transcripts with a personal computer. *Nurse Education Today*, **14**, 111–17.

Burnard, P. (1995) *Health Care Computing*, Chapman & Hall, London.

Burnard, P. (1995) Nurse educators' perceptions of reflection and reflective practice: a report of a descriptive study. *Journal of Advanced Nursing*, **21**, 1167–74.

Burnard, P. (1995) Writing for publication: a guide for those who must. *Nurse Education Today*, **15**, 117–20.

Burnard, P. and Chapman, C. (1993) *Professional and Ethical Issues in Nursing*, 2nd edn, Scutari, London.

Burnard, P. and Morrison, P. (1992) Students' and lecturers' preferred teaching strategies. *International Journal of Nursing Studies*, **29**(4), 345–53.

Burnard, P. and Morrison, P. (1994) *Nursing Research in Action: Developing Basic Skills*, 2nd edn, Macmillan, London.

Burrell, T. (1988) *Curriculum Design and Development: A Procedure Manual for Nurse Educators*, Prentice-Hall, Hemel Hempstead.

Byrne, S. (1991) Counselling – an essential nursing skill. *World of Irish Nursing*, **20**(4), 26–7.

Cameron, B.L. and Mitchell, A.M. (1993) Reflective peer journals: developing authentic nurses. *Journal of Advanced Nursing*, **18**(2), 290–7.

Carpio, B.A. and Majumdar, B. (1993) Experiential learning: an approach to transcultural education for nursing. *Journal of Transcultural Nursing*, **4**(2), 4–11.

Cartedge, G. and Milburn, J. (1995) *Teaching Social Skills to Children and Youth: Innovative Approaches*, Allyn & Bacon, Boston.

Clare, A. (1993) Communication in health. *European Journal of Disorders of Communication*, **28**, 1–12.

Clare, J. (1993) A challenge to the rhetoric of emancipation: recreating a professional culture. *Journal of Advanced Nursing*, **18**(7), 1033–8.

Clark, D. (1991) Guidance, counselling therapy: responses to marital problems 1950–90. *Sociological Review*, **39**, 765–98.

Clark, J.M., Hopper, L. and Jesson, A. (1991) Communication skills: progression to counselling. *Nursing Times*, **87**(8), 41–3.

Clarke, C. and Watson, D. (1991) Informal carers of the dementing elderly: a study of relationships. *Nursing Practice*, **4**(4), 17–21.

Clarke, L. (1989) Intervention and certainty in counselling literature Part 1. *Senior Nurse*, **9**(4), 18–19.

Clift, I. and Magee, T. (1992) Developing a new counselling course. *Nursing Standard*, **6**(18), 34–6.

Cohen-Cole, S. (ed.) (1991) *The Medical Interview: The Three-Function Approach*, Mosby Year Book, St Louis.

Collins, J. and Collins, M. (1992) *Social Skills Training and the Professional Helper*, Wiley, Chichester.

Cooley, E. (1994) Training an interdisciplinary team in communication and decision-making skills. *Small Group Research*. **25**, 5–25.

Cormier, L.S. (1987) *The Professional Counsellor: A Process Guide to Helping*, Prentice-Hall, Englewood Cliffs, New Jersey.

Cramer, D. (1992) *Personality and Psychotherapy: Theory, Practice and Research*, Open University Press, Buckingham.

Crandall, S. (1993) How expert clinical educators teach what they know. *Journal of Continuing Education in the Health Professions*, **13**(1), 85–98.

Crits-Christoph, P., Baranackie, K. and Kurcias, J. (1991) Meta-analysis of therapist effects in psychotherapy outcome studies, in *Psychological Testing*, 3rd edn, Harper & Row, New York.

Crute, V.C. *et al.* (1989) An evaluation of a communication skills course for health visitor students. *Journal of Advanced Nursing*, **14**(7), 546–52.

Cummings, J., Hansen, E. and Sillings, R. (1990) Teaching interviewing skills by interactive video: Intertalk. *Journal of School Psychology*, **28**, 3–96.

Curtis, T. and Kibler, S. (1990) Counselling in care. *Nursing Times*, **86**.

Daniel, C. (1992) Counselling sexual abuse survivors. *Nursing Standard*, **6**(46), 28–31.

Darbyshire, P. (1993) In the hall of mirrors ... reflective practice. *Nursing Times*, **89**(49), 26–9.

Darkenwald, G.G. and Merriam, S.B. (1982) *Adult Education: Foundations of Practice*, Harper & Row, New York.

Davidhizor, R. (1992) Interpersonal communication: a review of eye contact. *Infection Control and Hospital Epidemiology*, **13**, 222–5.

Davies, J.M. (1991) A behavioural model for counselling the nursing mother. Breastfeeding Review, **2**(4), 154–7.

Davis, B.D. and Burnard, P. (1992) Academic levels in nursing. *Journal of Advanced Nursing*, **17**, 1395–400.

Davison, J. (1992) Approach with care ... individual or group counselling. *Nursing Times*, **88**(8), pp. 38–9.

De Paulo, B.M. (1992) Nonverbal behaviour and self-presentation. *Psychological Bulletin*, **111**, 203–43.

De Vito, J.A. (1993) *Essentials of Human Communication*, Harper Collins, New York.

Denton, P.L. (1992) Teaching interpersonal skills with videotape ... to chronically ill psychiatric clients. *Occupational Therapy in Mental Health*, **2**(4), 17–34.

Derlega, V., Metts, S., Petronio, S. and Margulis, S. (1993) *Self-disclosure*, Sage, Newbury Park.

Dewing, J. (1990) Reflective practice ... within primacy nursing from individual and group viewpoints. *Senior Nurse*, **10**(10), 26–8.

Dickson, D., Saunders, C. and Stringer, M. (1993) *Rewarding People*, Routledge, London.

Dillard, J.P. (1995) Rethinking the study of fear appeals: an emotional perspective. *Communication Theory*, **4**, 295–323.

Diller, L. (1990) Fostering the interdisciplinary team, fostering research in a society in transition. *Archives of Physical Medicine and Rehabilitation*, **71**, 275–8.

Dillon, J. (1990) *The Practice of Questioning*, Routledge, London.

Docking, S. (1994) Accredited learning – the assessment procedure: how to complete the assessment for the reflective practice module. *Professional Nurse*, **9**(4), 244–6.

Dorn, F.J. (1984) *Counselling as Applied Social Psychology: An introduction to the social influence model*, Charles C Thomas, Springfield, Illinois.

Doust, M. (1991) Student nurses and counselling services. *Nursing Standard*, **5**(15/16), 35–7.

Dryden, W. and Feltham, C. (1994) *Developing Counsellor Training*, Sage, London.

Dryden, W. and Yankura, J. (1992) *Daring to Be Myself*, Open University Press, Buckingham.

Eckes, T. (1994) Features of men, features of women: assessing stereotypic beliefs about gender subtypes. *British Journal of Social Psychology*, **33**, 107–23.

Elliott, R. and Shapiro, D.A. (1992) Client and therapist as analysts of significant events, in *Psychotherapy Process Research: Paradigmatic and Narrative Approaches*, (eds S.G. Toukmanian and D.L. Rennie), Sage, London, pp. 163–86.

Ellis, A. (1983) How to deal with your most difficult client: you. *Journal of Rational-Emotive Therapy*, **3**(1), 3–8.

Ellis, A. and Dryden, W. (1987) The Practice of Rational-Emotive Therapy, Springer, New York.

Ellis, C. (1993) Incorporating the affective domain into staff development programs. *Journal of Nursing Staff Development*, **9**(3), 127–30.

Ellis, R. and Whittington, D. (eds) (1983) *New Directions in Social Skills Training*, Croom Helm, London.

Epstein, R., Campbell, C., Cohen-Cole, S. *et al.* (1993) Perspectives on patient-doctor communication. *Journal of Family Practice*, **37**, 377–88.

Evans, M.L. (1989) Simulations: their selection and use in developing nursing competencies. *Journal of Nursing Staff Development*, **5**(2), 65–9.

Eysenck, H.J. (1992) The outcome problem in psychotherapy, in *Psychotherapy and its Discontents*, (eds W. Dryden and C. Feltham), Open University Press, Buckingham, pp 100–23.

Farley, R.C. and Baker, A.J. (1987) Training on selected self-management techniques and the generalization and maintenance of interpersonal skills for registered nurse students. *Journal of Nursing Education*, **26**(3), 104–7.

Farrington, A. (1993) Intuition and expert clinical practice in nursing. *British Journal of Nursing*, **2**(4), 228–9.

Fedor, D., Rensvold, R. and Adams, S. (1992) An investigation of factors expected to affect feedback seeking: a longitudinal field study. *Personnel Psychology*, **45**, 779–805.

Feldman, R.S. and Rime, B. (eds) (1991) *Fundamentals of Nonverbal Behaviour*, Cambridge University Press, Cambridge.

Feltham, C. and Dryden, W. (1994) *Developing Counsellor Supervision*, Sage, London.

Ford, J. and Fisher, S. (1994) The transfer of safety training in work organisations: a systems perspective to continuous learning. *Occupational Medicine*, **9**, 241–59.

Forgas, J.P. (1994) The role of emotion in social judgments: an introductory review and an Affect Infusion Model. *Journal of Social Psychology*, **24**, 1–24.

Frederikson, L. and Bull, P. (1992) An appraisal of the current status of communication skills training in British medical schools. *Social Science and Medicine*, **34**, 515–22.

French, P. (1994) *Social Skills for Nursing Practice*, 2nd edn, Chapman & Hall, London.

French, P. and Cross, D. (1992) An interpersonal epistemological curriculum model for nurse education. *Journal of Advanced Nursing*, **17**(1), 83–9.

Frost, R., Benton, N. and Dowrick, P. (1990) Self-evaluation, videotape review and dysphoria. *Journal of Social and Clinical Psychology*, **9**, 367–74.

Galbraith, M. (ed.) (1990) *Adult Learning Methods: A Guide for Effective Instruction*, Krieger, Malabar, California.

Gallant, J., Thyer, B. and Bailey, J. (1991) Using bug-in-the-ear feedback in clinical supervision: preliminary evaluations. *Research on Social Work Practice*, **1**, 175–87.

Gamel, C., Davis, B.D. and Hengeveld, M. (1993) Nurses' provision of teaching and counselling on sexuality: review of the literature. *Journal of Advanced Nursing*, **18**(8), 1219–27.

Garavaglia, P. (1993) How to ensure transfer of training. *Training and Development*, **47**, 63–8.

Garfield, S.L. and Bergin, A.E. (1994) Introduction and historical overview in *Handbook of Psychotherapy and Behaviour Change*, 4th edn, (eds A.E. Bergin and S.L. Garfield), Wiley, Chichester, pp. 3–18.

Garko, M. (1992) Physician executives' use of influence strategies: gaining compliance from superiors who communicate in attractive and unattractive styles. *Health Communication*, **4**, 137–54.

Garrud, P. (1990) Counselling needs and experience of junior hospital doctors. *British Medical Journal*, **300**, 445–7.

Garvin, B.J. and Kennedy, C. (1990) Interpersonal communication between nurses and patients. *Annual Review of Nursing Research*, **8**, 213–34.

Gask, L., Goldberg, D. and Boardman, A. (1991) Training general practitioners to teach psychiatric interviewing skills: an evaluation of group training. *Medical Education*, **25**, 444–51.

Gaston, S. (1991) Sampling; an experiential learning activity. *Nurse Educator*, **16**(5), 4, 12.

Geldard, D. (1993) *Basic Personal Counselling*, 2nd edn, Prentice-Hall, Sydney.

Gelso, C. and Gassinger, R. (1990) Counselling psychology: theory and research on interventions. *Annual Review of Psychology*, **41**, 355–86.

General Medical Council (1993) *Tomorrow's Doctor: Recommendations on Undergraduate Medical Education*, General Medical Council, London.

Gershen, J. (1983) Use of experiential techniques in interpersonal skill training. *Journal of Dental Education*, **47**, 72–5.

Gibson, R.L. and Mitchell, M.H. (1986) *Introduction to Counselling and Guidance*, Collier Macmillan, London.

Gillam, T. (1993) Representational systems in counselling. *Nursing Standard*, **8**(10), 25–7.

Gist, M., Stevens, C. and Bavetta, A. (1991) The effects of self–efficacy and post-training intervention on the acquisition and maintenance of complex interpersonal skills. *Personnel Psychology*, **44**, 837–61.

Glueckauf, R.L. and Quittner, A.L. (1992) Assertiveness training for disabled adults in wheelchairs: self-report, role-play, and activity pattern outcomes. *Journal of Consulting and Clinical Psychology*, **60**, 419–25.

Goldfried, M.R., Greenberg, L.S. and Marmar, C. (1990) Individual psychotherapy: process and outcome. *Annual Review of Psychology*, **41**, 659–88.

Gordon, J. (1991) Measuring the goodness of training. *Training*, August, 19–25.

Gould, D. (1990) Empathy: a review of the literature with suggestions for an alternative research strategy. *Journal of Advanced Nursing*, **15**(10), 1167–74.

Gray, D. (1988) Counselling in general practice. *Journal of the Royal College of General Practitioners*, **38**, 50–1.

Greenberg, L.S. (1992) Task analysis: identifying components of interpersonal conflict resolution in *Psychotherapy Process Research: Paradigmatic and Narrative Approaches*, (eds S.G. Toukmanian and D.L. Rennie), Sage, London, pp. 22–50.

Greenberg, M.A. and Stone, A.A. (1992) Emotional disclosure about traumas and its relation to health: effects of previous disclosure and trauma severity. *Journal of Personality and Social Psychology*, **63**, 75–84.

Greenwood, J. (1993) Reflective practice: a critique of the work of Argyris and Schon. *Journal of Advanced Nursing*, **18**(8), 1183–7.

Greenwood, J. (1993) Some considerations concerning practice and feedback in nursing education. *Journal of Advanced Nursing*, **18**(12), 1999–2002.

Grencavage, L.N. and Norcross, J.C. (1990) Where are the commonalities among the therapeutic common factors? *Professional Psychology: Research and Practice*, **21**, 372–8.

Guccione, A.A. and DeMont, M.E. (1987) Interpersonal skills education in entry-level physical therapy programs. *Physical Therapy*, **67**(3), 388–93.

Guinn, C.A. (1992) Experiential learning: a 'real-world' introduction for baccalaureate nursing students. *Nurse Educator*, **17**(3), 31, 36.

Hadlow, J. and Pitts, M. (1991) The understanding of common health terms by doctors, nurses and patients. *Social Science and Medicine*, 32, 193–6.

Hamilton, M.A., Rouse, R.A. and Rouse, J. (1994) Dentist communication and patient utilization of dental services: anxiety inhibition and competence enhancement effects. *Health Communication*, **6**, 247–51.

Hargie, C., Dickson, D. and Tourish, D. (1994) Communication skills training (CST) and the radiography profession: a paradigm for training and development. *Research in Radiography*, **3**, 6–19.

Hargie, O., Saunders, C. and Dickson, D. (1994) *Social Skills in Interpersonal Communication*, 3rd edn, Routledge, London.

Hartley, P. (1993) *Interpersonal Communication*, Routledge, London.

Hasler, K. (1993) Bereavement counselling. *Nursing Standard*, **7**(40), 31–6.

Heath, R.L. and Bryant, J. (1992) *Human Communication Theory and Research: Concepts, Contexts and Challenges*, Lawrence Erlbaum Associates, Hillsdale, New Jersey.

Heppner, P.P., Kivlighan Jr., D.M. and Wampold, B.E. (1992) *Research Design in Counselling*, Brooks/Cole, Pacific Grove, California.

Hill, C.E. (1989) *Therapist Techniques and Client Outcomes: Eight Cases of Brief Psychotherapy*, Sage, London.

Hill, C.E. (1991) Almost everything you ever wanted to know about how to do process research on counselling and psychotherapy but didn't know who to ask, in *Research in Counselling*, (eds C.E. Watkins and L.J. Schneider), Lawrence Erlbaum Associates, Hillsdale, New Jersey, pp. 85–118.

Hill, C.E. and Corbett, M.M. (1993) A perspective on the history of process and outcome research in counselling psychology. *Journal of Counselling Psychology*, **32**, 3–22.

Holli, B. and Calabrese, R. (1991) *Communication and Education Skills: The Dietician's Guide*, Lea & Febiger, Philadelphia.

Hopper, E. (1991) Shattered dreams ... counselling work with bereaved parents. *Nursing Standard*, **6**(4), 20–1.

Hummert, M.L., Wiemann, J.W. and Nussbaum, J.F. (eds) (1994) *Interpersonal Communication in Older Adulthood: Interdisciplinary Theory and Research*, Sage, Thousand Oaks, California.

Ivey, A.E. (1987) *Counselling and Psychotherapy: Skills, Theories and Practice*, Prentice-Hall International, London.

Jackson, L.D. (1992) Information complexity and medical communication: the effects of technical language and amount of information in a medical message. *Health Communication*, **4**, 197–210.

Jackson, L.D. (1994) Maximising treatment adherence among back-pain patients: an experimental study of the effects of physician-related cues in written medical messages. *Health Communication*, **6**, 173–91.

Jacob, M.R. (1988) Putting research into practice: the impact of interpersonal skills training on responses to patients' emotional concerns by nursing staff in a general hospital. *Florida Nurse*, **36**(9), 18.

Jarvis, P. (1983) *Professional Education*, Croom Helm, London.

Jarvis, P. (1987) Meaningful and meaningless experience: towards an understanding. *Adult Education Quarterly*, **37**, 3.

Jeavons, B. (1991) Developing counselling skills. *Nursing (London), The Journal of Clinical Practice Education and Management*, **4**(38), 28–9.

Johns, C. (1993) On becoming effective in taking ethical action. *Journal of Clinical Nursing*, **2**(5), 307–12.

Johns, C. (1993) Professional supervision. *Journal of Nursing Management*, **1**(1), 9–18.

Jonassen, D. and Grabowski, B. (1993) *Handbook of Individual Differences, Learning, and Instruction*, Lawrence Erlbaum Associates, Hillsdale, New Jersey.

Jones, A. (1991) The path towards a common goal: structuring the counselling process. *Professional Nurse*, **6**(6), 302, 304–6.

Jones, A. (1992) Confronting the inevitable … counselling … a patient. *Nursing Standard*, **6**(46), 54–6.

Jones, A. (1993) A first step in effective communication: providing a supportive environment for counselling in hospital. *Professional Nurse*, **8**(8), 501–5.

Jones, C. (1990) All you ever wanted to know about … counselling. *Nursing Times*, **10**, 55–8.

Jones, J. (1991) Therapeutic use of metaphor. *Nursing Standard*, **6**(11), 30–2.

Jupp, J. and Griffiths, M. (1990) Self-concept changes in shy, socially isolated adolescents following social skills training emphasising role-plays. *Australian Psychologist*, **25**, 165–77.

Kelly, C., Moran, T. and Myatt, P. (1994) Conversion disorder, sexual abuse and interprofessional communication – some lessons to be re-learned. *Irish Journal of Psychological Medicine*, **11**, 135–7.

Kendrick, T. and Freeling, P. (1993) A communication skills course for preclinical students: evaluation of general practice based teaching using group methods. *Medical Education*, **27**, 211–17.

Kernis, M. and Sun, C.R. (1994) Narcissism and reactions to interpersonal feedback. *Journal of Advanced Nursing*, **18**, 1324–30.

Knapp, M. and Hall, J. (1992) *Nonverbal Communication in Human Interaction*, Holt, Rinehart, and Winston, New York.

Kreps, G. and Kunimoto, E.N. (1994) *Effective Communication in Multicultural Health Care Settings*, Sage, Thousand Oaks, California.

Laird, D. (1991) *Approaches to Training and Development*, Addison-Wesley, New York.

Laker, D. (1990) Dual dimensionality of training transfer. *Human Resource Development Quarterly*, **1**, 209–23.

Lambert, B. (1995) Directness and deference in pharmacy students' messages to physicians. *Social Science and Medicine*, **40**, 5456.

Lang, G. and van der Molen, H. (1990) *Personal Conversations: Roles and Skills for Counsellors*, Routledge, London.

Lee, J. and Whitford, M. (1992) Effects of performance feedback on teachers' self-evaluations. *Psychological Reports*, **71**, 323–31.

Lewis, J. (1994) Patient views on quality care in general practice: literature review. *Social Science and Medicine*, **39**, 655–70.

Lierman, B. (1994) How to develop a training simulation. *Training and Development*, **48**, 50–2.

Lister, P. (1989) Experiential learning and the benefits of journal work. *Senior Nurse*, **9**(6), 20–1.

Lopez, K.A. (1983) Role modelling interpersonal skills with beginning nursing students: gestalt techniques. *Journal of Nursing Education*, **22**(3), 119–22.

Macaskill, N. and Macaskill, A. (1992) Psychotherapists-in-training evaluate their personal therapy: results of a UK survey. *British Journal of Psychotherapy*, **9**(2), 133–8.

Magill, R. (1993) *Motor Learning: Concepts and Applications*, W.C. Brown, Dubuque, Iowa.

Magill, R. (1994) The influence of augmented feedback on skill learning depends on characteristics of the skill and learner. *Quest*, **46**, 27–31.

Maguire, P. (1991) Managing difficult communication tasks, in *Developing Communication Skills in Medicine*, (ed. R. Corney), Routledge, London.

Maguire, P. and Faulkner, A. (1988) Improving the counselling skills of doctors and nurses in cancer care. *British Medical Journal*, **297**, 847–9.

Mahrer, A. and Nadler, W. (1986) 'Good moments in psychotherapy: a preliminary review, a list and some promising research avenues. *Journal of Consulting and Clinical Psychology*, **54**(1), 10–15.

Makely, S. (1990) Methods for teaching effective patient communication techniques to radiography students. *Radiography Today*, **56**, 14–15.

Mander, R. (1992) See how they learn: experience as the basis of practice. *Nurse Education Today*, **121**, 3–10.

Marte, A.L. (1991) Experiential learning strategies for promoting positive staff attitudes toward the elderly. *Journal of Continuing Education in Nursing*, **22**(2), 73–7.

Martin, E., Russell, D., Goodwin, S. *et al.* (1991) Why patients consult and what happens when they do. *British Medical Journal*, **303**, 289–92.

Marx, R. and Ivey, A. (1988) Communication skills programmes that last: face to face and relapse prevention. *International Journal for the Advancement of Counselling*, **11**, 135–51.

Mason, P. (1992) Allowing for loss … bereavement counselling. *Nursing Times*, **88**(2), 14–15.

Matthews, A. (1993) Biases in processing emotional information. *The Psychologist*, **6**, 493–9.

Maxwell, M., Dickson, D. and Saunders, C. (1991) An evaluation of communication skills training for physiotherapy students. *Medical Teacher*, **13**, 333–8.

May, C. (1990) Research on nurse–patient relationships: problems of theory, problems of practice. *Journal of Advanced Nursing*, **15**, 307–15.

McCartan, P.J. and Hargie, O. (1990) Assessing assertive behaviour in student nurses: a comparison of assertion measures. *Journal of Advanced Nursing*, **15**, 1370–6.

McCaugherty, D. (1991) The use of a teaching model to promote reflection and the experiential integration of theory and practice in first-year student-nurses: an action research study. *Journal of Advanced Nursing*, **16**(5), 534–43.

McGregor, J. (1993) Effectiveness of role playing and anti-racial teaching in reducing student prejudice. *Journal of Educational Research*, **86**, 215–26.

McLeod, J. (1994) The research agenda for counselling. *Counselling*, **5**(1), 41–3.

McLeod, J. (1994) Issues in the organisation of counselling: learning from NMGC. *British Journal of Guidance and Counselling*, **22**(2), 163–74.

Mcmanus, I.C., Vincent, C.A., Thom, S. and Kidd, J. (1993) Teaching communication skills to clinical students. *British Medical Journal*, **306**, 1322–7.

McMillan, I. (1991) A listening ear … telephone counselling. *Nursing Times*, **87**(6), 30–1.

McWilliams, S. (1991) Affective changes following severe head injury as perceived by patients and relatives. *British Journal of Occupational Therapy*, **54**(7), 246–8.

Meeuwesen, L., Schaap, C. and van der Staak, C. (1991) Verbal analysis of doctor–patient communication. *Social Science and Medicine*, **32**, 1143–50.

Meharg, S. and Woltersdorf, M. (1990) Therapeutic use of videotape self-modelling: a review. *Advances in Behaviour Research and Therapy*, **32**, 85–99.

Melby, V. (1992) Counselling of patients with HIV related diseases: what is the role of the nurse? *Journal of Clinical Nursing*, **1**(1), 39–45.

Meredith, P. (1993) Patient satisfaction with communication in general surgery. *Social Science and Medicine*, 37, 591–602.

Merriam, S. (1984) Mentors and protégés: a critical review of the literature. *Adult Education Quarterly*, **33**(3), 161–73.

Mezeiro, J. (1981) A critical theory of adult learning and education. *Adult Education*, **32**(1), 3–24.

Millar, R., Crute, V. and Hargie, O. (1992) *Professional Interviewing*, Routledge, London.

Millar, R., Goldman, E., Bor, R. and Scher, I. (1992) Counselling in terminal care. *Nursing Standard*, **6**(26), 52–5.

Miller, G. and Stiff, J. (1993) *Deceptive Communication*, Sage, Newbury Park.

Miller, R. (1993) Bereavement counselling in HIV disease. *Nursing Standard*, **7**(39), 48–51.

Mills, G. and Pace, R. (1989) What effects do practice and video feedback have on the development of interpersonal communication skills? *Journal of Business Communication*, **26**, 159–76.

Mocker, D.W. and Spear, G.E. (1982) *Lifelong Learning: Formal, Non-formal and Self-Directed*, The ERIC Clearinghouse on Adult Career and Vocational Education, New York.

Moore, E.R., Bianchi-Gray, M. and Stephens, P. (1992) A community hospital-based breastfeeding counselling service. *Breastfeeding Review*, **2** (6), 264–70.

Morrison, P., Burnard, P. and Hackett, P. (1991) A smallest space analysis of nurses' perceptions of their interpersonal skills. *Counselling Psychology Quarterly*, **4**(2/3), 119–25.

Morrow, N. and Hargie, O. (1985) Interpersonal communication: questioning skills. *Pharmacy Update*, **1**, 255–7.

Morrow, N. and Hargie, O. (1994) Communication skills and health promotion. *Pharmaceutical Journal*, 253, 311–13.

Morsund, J. (1985) *The Process of Counselling and Therapy*, Prentice-Hall, Englewood Cliffs, New Jersey.

Murgatroyd, S. (1986) *Counselling and Helping*, British Psychological Society and Methuen, London.

Murgatroyd, S. and Woolfe, R. (1982) *Coping with Crisis – Understanding and Helping Persons in Need*, Harper & Row, London.

Myerscough, P.R. (1989) *Talking With Patients: A Basic Clinical Skill*, Oxford Medical Publications, Oxford.

Nadler, L. (ed.) (1984) *The Handbook of Human Resource Development*, Wiley, New York.

Napier, R.W. and Gershenfeld, M.K. (1993) *Group Theory and Experience*, Houghton Mifflin, Boston.

Nelson-Jones, R. (1988) *Practical Counselling and Helping Skills: Helping Clients to Help*, Cassell, London.

Nelson-Jones, R. (1991) *Lifeskills: A Handbook*, Cassell, London.

Nesbitt, M.L. (1990) Failing to communicate. *Journal of the Medical Defence Union*, **6**, 49.

Newell, R. (1992) Anxiety, accuracy and reflection: the limits of professional development. *Journal of Advanced Nursing*, **17**(11), 1326–33.

Newell, R. (1994) *Interviewing Skills for Nurses and Other Health Care Professionals. A Structured Approach*, Routledge, London.

Newell, R. and Dryden, W. (1991) Clinical problems: an introduction to the cognitive-behavioural approach, in *Clinical Problems: A Cognitive-Behavioural Approach*, (eds W. Dryden and R. Rentoul), Routledge, London.

Nkowane, A.M. (1993) Breaking the silence: the need for counselling of HIV/AIDS patients. *International Nursing Review*, **40**(1), 17–20, 24.

Noble, C. (1991) Are nurses good patient educators? *Journal of Advanced Nursing*, **16**, 1185–9.

Noe, R. (1986) Trainees' attributes and attitudes: neglected influences on training effectiveness. *Academy of Management Review*, **11**, 736–49.

Noe, R., Sears, J. and Fullenkamp, A. (1990) Relapse training: does it influence trainees' post-training behaviour and cognitive strategies? *Journal of Business and Psychology*, **4**, 317–28.

Norris, J. (1986) Teaching communication skills: effects of two methods of instruction and selected learner characteristics. *Journal of Nurse Education*, **25**, 102–6.

Nyatanga, L. (1989) Experiential taxonomy and experiential learning. *Senior Nurse*, **9**(8), 24–7.

Nytanga, L. (1989) Social skills training: some ideas on its origin, nature and application. *Nurse Education Today*, **9**(1), 56–63.

O'Hair, D. and Friedrich, G.W. (1992) *Strategic Communication in Business and the Professions*, Houghton Mifflin, Boston.

Ohlsen, A.M., Horne, A.M. and Lawe, C.F. (1988) *Group Counselling*, Holt, Rinehart and Winston, New York.

Olson, J.K. and Iwasiw, C.L. (1987) Effects of a training model on active listening skills of post-RN students. *Journal of Nursing Education*, **26**(3), 104–7.

Omer, H. and Dar, R. (1992) Changing trends in three decades of psychotherapy research: the flight from theory into pragmatics. *Journal of Consulting and Clinical Psychology*, **60**, 88–93.

Open University Coping With Crisis Group (1987) *Running Workshops: A Guide for Trainers in the Helping Professions*, Croom Helm, London.

Parathian, A. and Taylor, F. (1993) Can we insulate trainee nurses from exposure to bad practice? A study of role play in communicating bad news to patients. *Journal of Advanced Nursing*, **18**, 801–7.

Parrott, R. (1994) Exploring family practitioners' and patients' information exchange about prescribed medications: implications for practitioners' interviewing and patients' understanding. *Health Communication*, **6**, 267–80.

Parry, G. (1992) Improving psychotherapy services: applications of research, audit and evaluation. *British Journal of Clinical Psychology*, **31**, 3–19.

Paunonen, M. (1991) Testing a model for counsellor training in three public health-care organisations. *Nurse Education Today*, **11**(4), 270–7.

Perloff, R. (1993) *The Dynamics of Persuasion*, Lawrence Erlbaum Associates, Hillsdale, New Jersey.

Phillips, J. (1993) Counselling and the nurse. *British Journal of Theatre Nursing*, **2**(10), 13(4).

Pringle, M. and Stewart-Evans, C. (1990) Does awareness of being video recorded affect doctors' consultation behaviour? *British Journal of General Practice*, **40**, 455–8.

Pulsford, D. (1993) Reducing the threat: an experiential exercise to introduce role play to student nurses. *Nurse Education Today*, **13**(2), 145–8.

Pulsford, D. (1993) The reluctant participant in experiential learning. *Nurse Education Today*, **13**(2), 139–44.

Quigley, B. and Nyquist, J. (1992) Using video technology to provide feedback to students in performance courses. *Communication Education*, **41**, 324–34.

Ramos, M.C. (1992) The nurse–patient relationship: theme and variations. *Journal of Advanced Nursing*, **17**, 496–506.

Reardon, K. (1991) *Persuasion in Practice*, Sage, Newbury Park.

Reddy, M. (1987) *The Manager's Guide to Counselling at Work,* Methuen, London.

Rees, A.M. (1993) Communication in the physician–patient relationship. *Bulletin of the Medical Library Association*, **81**, 1–10.

Reid, B. (1993) 'But we're doing it already!' Exploring a response to the concept of reflective practice in order to improve its facilitation. *Nurse Education Today*, **13**(4), 305–9.

Reid, W. and Long, A. (1993) The role of the nurse providing therapeutic care for the suicidal patient. *Journal of Advanced Nursing*, **18**(13), 69–76.

Ricketts, T. (1993) Therapist self-disclosure in behavioural psychotherapy. *British Journal of Nursing*, **2**(13), 667–71.

Ridderikhoff, J. (1993) Information exchange in a patient physician encounter. A quantitative approach. *Methods in Information and Medicine*, **32**, 73–8.

Robotham, A. (1992) The use of credit and experiential learning in nurse education. Exciting opportunities for student and tutor alike. *Nurse Education Today*, **11**(6), 448–53.

Roffers, T., Cooper, B. and Sultanoff, S. (1988) Can counsellor trainees apply their skills in actual client interviews? *Journal of Counselling and Development*, **66**, 385–8.

Rolfe, G. (1990) The assessment of therapeutic attitudes in the psychiatric setting. *Journal of Advanced Nursing*, **15**(5), 564–70.

Rolfe, G. (1990) The role of clinical supervision in the education of student psychiatric nurses: a theoretical approach. *Nurse Education Today*, **10**(3), 193–7.

Rolfe, G. (1993) Closing the theory–practice gap: a model of nursing praxis. *Journal of Clinical Nursing*, **2**(2), 89–93.

Rosenfarb, I., Hayes S. and Linehan, M. (1989) Instructions and experiential feedback in the treatment of social skills deficits in adults. *Psychotherapy*, **26**, 242–51.

Ross, F.M., Bower, P.J. and Sibbald, B.S. (1994) Practice nurses: characteristics, workload and training needs. *British Journal of General Practice*, **44**, 15–18.

Rowland, N., Irving, J. and Maynard, A. (1989) Can general practitioners counsel? *Journal of the Royal College of General Practitioners*, **39**, 118–20.

Rugg, D.L. *et al.* (1992) Evaluating the CDC programme for HIV counselling and testing. *International Nursing Review*, **39**(5), 157–60.

Sampson Jr, J.P. (1991) The place of the computer in counselling research, in *Research in Counselling*, (eds C.E. Watkins and L.J. Schneider), Lawrence Erlbaum Associates, Hillsdale, New Jersey, pp. 261–86.

Sanson-Fisher, R., Redman, R., Walsh, R. *et al.* (1991) Training medical practitioners in information transfer skills: the new challenge. *Medical Education*, **25**, 322–33.

Satow, A. and Evans, M. (1983) *Working with Groups*, Tacade, Manchester.

Schneider, D.E. and Tucker, R. (1992) Measuring communicative satisfaction in doctor–patient relations: the doctor–patient inventory. *Health Communication*, **4**, 19–28.

Seale, C. (1992) Community nurses and the care of the dying. *Social Science and Medicine*, **34**, 375–82.

Sellick, K. (1991) Nurses' interpersonal behaviours and the development of helping skills. *International Journal of Nursing Studies*, **28**, 3–11.

Shapiro, S.B. (1985) An empirical analysis of operating values in humanistic education. *Journal of Humanistic Psychology*, **25** (1), 94–108.

Shropshire, C.O. (1981) Group experiential learning in adult education. *Journal of Continuing Education in Nursing*, **12**(6), 5–9.

Slater, J. (1990) Effecting personal effectiveness: assertiveness training for nurses. *Journal of Advanced Nursing*, **15**, 337–56.

Sleight, P. (1995) Teaching communication skills: part of medical education? *Journal of Human Hypertension*, **9**, 67–9.

Sloan, D., Donnelly, M., Johnson, S. *et al.* (1994) Assessing surgical residents' and medical students' interpersonal skills. *Journal of Surgical Research*, **57**, 613–18.

Snyder, M. (1987) *Public Appearances, Private Realities: The Psychology of Self-monitoring*, Freeman, New York.

Snyder, M. (1993) Critical thinking: a foundation for consumer-focused care. *Journal of Continuing Education in Nursing*, **24**(5), 206–10.

Speck, P. (1992) Managing the boundaries ... using our counselling skills to help a colleague or a student can create more problems. *Nursing Times*, **88**(32), 22.

Spitzberg, B. and Cupach, W. (1989) *Handbook of Interpersonal Competence Research*, Springer, New York.

Steenbarger, B.N. (1992) Toward science–practice integration in brief counselling and psychotherapy. *Counselling Psychologist*, **20**, 403–50.

Stiles, W.B., Elliott, R., Llewellyn, S. *et al.* (1990) Assimilation of problematic experiences by clients in psychotherapy. *Psychotherapy*, **27**, 411–20.

Stitch, T.F. (1983) Experiential therapy. *Journal of Experiential Education*, **5**(3), 23–30.

Street, R.L. (1992) Analyzing communication in medical consultations. Do behavioural measures correspond to patients' perceptions? *Medical Care*, **30**, 976–88.

Stricker, G. and Fisher, M. (eds) (1990) *Self-disclosure in the Therapeutic Relationship*, Plenum Press, New York.

Stroebe, W. (1994) Why groups are less effective than their members: on personality losses in idea-generating groups. *BPS Social Psychology Section Newsletter*, **31**, 4–20.

Talbot, C. (1992) Evaluation and validation: a mixed approach. *Journal of European Industrial Training*, **16**, 22–32.

Tannenbaum, S. and Yukl, G. (1992) Training and development in work organisations. *Annual Review of Psychology*, **43**, 399–441.

Thomas, P. (1993) An exploration of patients' perceptions of counselling with particular reference to counselling within general practice. *Counselling*, **4**, 24–30.

Thompson, A.N. (1992) Can communication skills be assessed independently of their context? *Medical Education*, **26**, 364–7.

Thorne, B. and Dryden, W. (1993) *Counselling: Interdisciplinary Perspectives*, Open University Press, Buckingham.

Thorne, P. (1991) Assessment of prior experiential learning. *Nursing Standard*, **6**(10), 32–4.

Tittmar, H., Hargie, O. and Dickson, D. (1978) The moulding of health visitors: the evolved role played by mini-training. *Health Visitor Journal*, **51**, 130–6.

Tourish, D. and Hargie, O. (1993) Quality assurance and internal organisational communications. *International Journal of Health Care Quality Assurance*, **6**, 22–8.

Turner, J.C. (1991) *Social Influence*, Open University Press, Buckingham.

Weldon, E. and Weingart, L. (1993) Group goals and group performance. *British Journal of Social Psychology*, **32**, 307–34.

Wetchler, J. and Vaughan, K. (1991) Perceptions of primary supervisors' interpersonal skills: a critical incident analysis. *Contemporary Family Therapy*, **13**, 61–8.

White, J., Levinson,W. and Roter, D. (1994) Oh by the way … . The closing moments of the medical visit. *Journal of General and Internal Medicine*, **9**, 24–8.

Whitehouse, C. (1991) The teaching of communication skills in United Kingdom medical schools. *Medical Education*, **25**, 11–18.

Wilke, H.A.M. and Meertens, R.W. (1994) *Group Performance*, Routledge, London.

Wilkinson, S. (1991) Factors which influence how nurses communicate with cancer patients. *Journal of Advanced Nursing*, **16**, 677–88.

Wilmot, W. (1995) *Relational Communication*, McGraw-Hill, New York.

Wilson, L.K. and Gallois, C. (1993) *Assertion and its Social Context*, Pergamon, Oxford.

Wolvin, A. and Coakley, C. (eds) (1993) *Perspectives on Listening*, Ablex, Norwood, New Jersey.

Wright, J. (1991) Counselling at the cultural interface: is getting back to roots enough? *Journal of Advanced Nursing*, **16**(1), 92–100.

Wyatt, P. (1993) The role of nurses in counselling the terminally ill patient. *British Journal of Nursing*, **2**(14), 701–4.

Yoder, D., Hugenberg, L. and Wallace, S. (1993) *Creating Competent Communication*, W.C. Brown, Dubuque, Iowa.

Zebrowitz, L.A. (1990) *Social Perception*, Open University, Milton Keynes.

Zimbardo, P. and Leippe, M. (1991) *The Psychology of Attitude Change and Social Influence*, McGraw-Hill, New York.

Index